Overcoming Depression and Low Mood
A Five Areas Approach

Overcoming Depression and Low Mood

A Five Areas Approach

Fourth Edition

Dr Chris Williams MBChB BSc MMedSC MD
FRCPsych BABCP Accredited CBT practitioner
Senior Lecturer and Honorary Consultant
Psychiatrist, Section of Psychological Medicine,
Faculty of Medicine, University of Glasgow, UK

Helping you to help yourself
www.livinglifetothefull.com
www.fiveareas.com

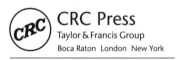

CRC Press
Taylor & Francis Group
Boca Raton London New York

CRC Press is an imprint of the
Taylor & Francis Group, an **informa** business

CRC Press
Taylor & Francis Group
6000 Broken Sound Parkway NW, Suite 300
Boca Raton, FL 33487-2742

© 2015 by Chris Williams
CRC Press is an imprint of Taylor & Francis Group, an Informa business

No claim to original U.S. Government works

Printed on acid-free paper
Version Date: 20141106

International Standard Book Number-13: 978-1-4441-8377-1 (Paperback)

Visit the Taylor & Francis Web site at
http://www.taylorandfrancis.com

and the CRC Press Web site at
http://www.crcpress.com

Contents

Buying the books in bulk: Bulk copies of the book are available at discounted rates direct from the publisher and also from **www.fiveareas.com**

Introduction

Welcome to the fourth edition of *Overcoming Depression and Low Mood: A Five Areas Approach*. It's been good to hear from so many people who have benefitted from using this resource. Hopefully, whether you are a practitioner or a member of the public wanting to use these resources in your own life, you'll find at least something that helps.

This book teaches important information about how low mood can affect your life. It aims to help you work out why you sometimes feel low, anxious, angry or guilty. It also teaches proven practical skills to help change how you feel.

By using the clearly described practical tools in these workbooks, you can make helpful changes to your life.

Who are the workbooks for?

You may be using the workbooks for yourself, or perhaps you are a close friend or family member wanting to know more about depression and low mood and how to help. Many healthcare practitioners also use the workbooks and they are widely used across a range of countries with tens of thousands of people who have benefitted from this approach.

The course can be used by people with problems ranging from mild distress through to more severe depression. The key thing is that you feel **able** to use the materials and **want** to use this approach.

Using the workbooks

Picking the right time to do the course is important. For example, if your concentration, energy or motivation levels are far lower than usual, you may find it very hard to keep your mind on things or to make changes. Other approaches such as anti-depressant medications may be more appropriate first – or can be used alongside this approach. If you find that you struggle to use the workbooks, or you feel worse as you work through them, please discuss this with your doctor or other healthcare practitioner. The course is not meant to replace getting the right level of support for more severe mental health problems.

Which workbook should you use first?

There is no right or wrong way to use the workbooks. Many people find it helpful to first read the two workbooks in Part 1 (*Starting out* and *Understanding why you feel as you do*). This is because these workbooks give you an overview of the approach.

Working through these workbooks will also help you to decide which of the *Making Changes* workbooks in Part 2 of the book you should read. You can use as many or as few workbooks in the course as you wish. You will feel most motivated to try to make changes if you use the workbooks that tackle problems you have noticed in your life and that you yourself want to change.

There is no right or wrong choice of workbooks to use, or a set course you must complete. The key to creating change in your life is **using** the workbooks that address problems relevant to you, and **putting what you learn into practice**.

Getting support from others

It can be hard making changes when you feel low. Many people start off trying to improve things with lots of motivation. But part of feeling low is that it's easy to get discouraged or talk ourselves out of change. That's entirely normal and is very human. (Think how hard people find it to keep New Year resolutions even when they aren't feeling low!).

Time and time again people using resources like this have found the benefits of working with someone else to support and encourage them when things feel hard. We therefore suggest that you partner up with someone to help you as you use the course, for example, a health or social services worker, your doctor, a voluntary sector worker or a trusted family member or friend.

The amount of support can be quite short – perhaps just 20 to 30 minutes over say four to six weeks. The important thing is to have someone else there, helping you, discussing ways of getting round possible blocks to change, and, of course, to say well done when things move forward.

A word of encouragement

Depression affects lots of people at some time in their lives. Fortunately, it has now become clear that by changing certain thoughts and behaviour patterns you can greatly improve how you feel. The content of these workbooks is based on the cognitive behavioural therapy (CBT; a kind of talking treatment) approach. The developers of CBT have found many effective ways of tackling the common symptoms and problems people face when feeling low.

This course is written in a way that clearly explains what to do, so that you can test the effect of these different suggestions in your own life. The workbooks aim to help you to **regain a sense of control** over how you feel.

The course does work

Research has been done involving people who used a previous edition of this book. The research found that, compared with people receiving usual care for depression, people using the workbooks with support:

- On average improved far more.

- Felt better and were more active.

- These benefits were present at both four and 12 months later.

The course can make a big difference if you can commit to using it. Having someone else to encourage you is also important.

International use of this approach

This course is widely used and recommended by professionals across the world.

- It was one of the first 100 recommended books to receive the ABCT (Association for Behavioral and Cognitive Therapies) seal of approval – a leading North American organization for Cognitive Behavioural Therapy.

- In the UK, the *Overcoming depression and low mood* book, and the companion book *Overcoming anxiety: a five areas approach* are both named among the 30 books chosen to be made available in every library across England as part of the national healthy reading Book Prescription Scheme.

- In Scotland, people can self-refer to receive free copies of the resources with phone-based support from NHS24 (the NHS Living Life Service).

- In England, the book and companion anxiety book are both recommended as resources in the Improving Access to Psychological Therapies (IAPT) courses.

- Well over 200,000 people have signed up for free online training using this course.

Overall, many people have been helped by this approach. But can it be useful for you?

Making a commitment

Sometimes making changes is easier said (or written) than done. All of us feel discouraged and overwhelmed from time to time. This is even more likely in times of low or anxious mood.

Therefore, **I would like to encourage you to try to make a commitment to use this course** and to keep at it even if you feel discouraged or stuck for a time. Set small goals and aim to move things forward step-by-step by focusing on just one workbook at a time. Be realistic. Bear in mind your motivation and energy levels so that you don't try to do more than you can at one time. This will help you to get as much from the course as you can at the moment.

The *Starting out* workbook gives some suggestions of how you can **pace things**, and also some suggestions of what to do if you are struggling.

Online resources

Three online resources are available to support users of the course:

1. **www.llttf.com (www.livinglifetothefull.com; Twitter @llttfnews).** This popular resource is designed to support readers of this course. There's also a popular forum where you can make comments, or ask questions of other people using the same course.

2. **www.llttf.com/shop for resources and books (for members of the public)**

3. **www.fiveareas.com (Twitter icon @fiveareas for practitioner support and training). This dedicated site is aimed at practitioners and points to the whole range of Five Areas resources, including books, handouts, training courses, translations, accessible versions, and more.**

Limited licence to use

Permission is given for limited copying of this book by the purchaser where this is for use in the normal course of the purchaser's business within the free-access healthcare industry and within small independent private healthcare clinics in relation to training and for client consultations. This permission extends to providing copies of the relevant part or parts of the book to a patient where relevant to a particular consultation.

This permission does not allow copying or use by other healthcare professionals and therefore each practitioner in a clinical service using this book must have his or her own purchased copy. Nor does this permission extend to any purchaser working for or within a large commercial organization, including but not limited to employment assistance programmes, health maintenance companies and insurance organizations. Such a purchaser or practitioner is not entitled to copy or otherwise use the book to assist members of any such organization unless a commercial licence has been obtained from the publishers.

Training

Training courses for practitioners are available. Contact us at events@fiveareas.com or alternatively visit **www.fiveareas.com/training.**

Acknowledgments

The illustrations in the workbooks have been produced by Keith Chan, kchan75@ hotmail.com.

The terms LLTTF and Five Areas are registered trademarks of Five Areas Resources Ltd. The *Planner* and *Review sheets*, and *Plan, Do, Review* model are reproduced from the Living Life to the Full course courtesy of Five Areas Resources Ltd© (2009–2013).

It's likely you'll find some parts of the course help more, and others less. If you have comments or suggested changes please do let me know via feedback@fiveareas. com and this really helps shape future content.

Finally, I hope the course proves helpful.

Dr Chris Williams
MBChB BSc MMedSc MD FRCPsych Hon Fellow BABCP
January 2014

Part 1
Understanding why you feel as you do

Starting out ... and how to keep going if you feel stuck

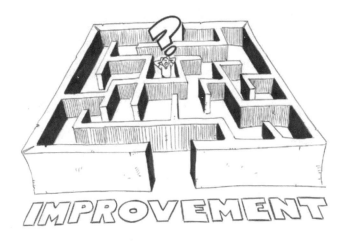

www.llttf.com or www.livinglifetothefull.com 🅣 @llttfnews (public)

www.fiveareas.com 🅣 @fiveareas (practitioners)

🅕 www.llttf.com/facebook

Dr Chris Williams

overcoming
depression and low mood
a five areas approach

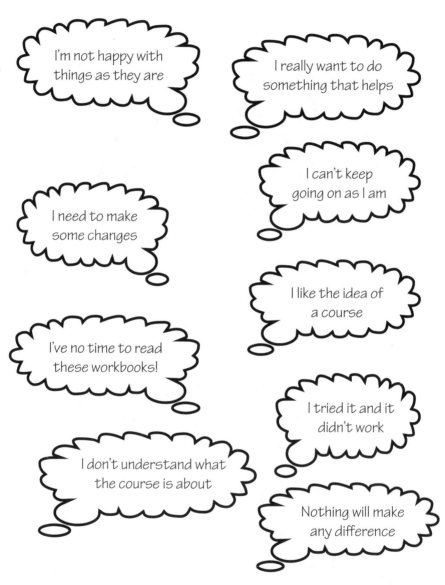

Are you feeling like this?

If so... this course is for you.

What you will learn:

- How to get the most out of this course.
- Make a clear but flexible plan of when to use this and the other workbooks.
- Discover how to overcome common blocks to change.

About the course

The workbooks in this course aim to help you understand why you feel as you do. They will teach you important life skills that will help you to turn the corner.

Why should you use these workbooks?

People use these workbooks because they want to make changes in their lives. **You, the reader, are in control** – and you can work on things at a time that suits you. Time and time again, people are surprised to see the amount of change they can make themselves using a structured approach.

These workbooks use an approach called cognitive behavioural therapy (CBT, a kind of talking treatment). Don't worry though – there won't be any more jargon like that in the rest of the course. Research has shown that self-help materials based on the CBT approach work well for problems such as depression and anxiety. Research on this book has also shown that it works very well as a treatment for depression. People using the book felt less depressed and were more able to live their lives as they wanted. This is why this book is one of only 30 books to be chosen to be included in every public library in England as part of the national Books on Prescription scheme.

Reference

www.plosone.org/article/info%3Adoi%2F10.1371%2Fjournal.pone.0052735
www.bbc.co.uk/news/health-21083458

Getting going

Well done! You've done something that quite a few people struggle to do – **you're still reading**.

It can sometimes seem really hard starting to change. Have you ever bought or been given a book or a DVD and never even opened it or even taken the wrapper off? Using this course is no different. In fact, in some ways it's harder because it's not a book that's there for entertainment. Instead these are workbooks which aim to help you to change how you feel.

What should I read first?

People usually start by working through these two workbooks:

● This one – *Starting out... and how to keep going if you feel stuck*

● And then *Understanding why you feel as you do.*

They will help you work out how your low mood is affecting you and help you decide which other workbooks to use.

> **KEY POINT**
> Choose the workbooks **you** want to work on – making sure they deal with the problems/difficulties **you** are facing.

Developing a routine

Routines can be powerful. For example, if you are used to having a snack while you watch television, sometimes just sitting in the same chair can make you feel hungry!

In the same way, you might wish to set aside a particular place to complete the workbooks. For example, sit on a chair at the kitchen table with a pen and some blank paper to jot down ideas as you read. Plan enough time so that you can get really involved in the workbook – preferably half an hour or so, if you have sufficient energy and concentration for this. If you have others around you, like young children who might interrupt, try to choose a time when they are asleep or away at nursery or school. Or see if a friend or relative could take them for a time while you work on the course.

Getting into the mood: doing something physical can help you get started

You may feel physically and mentally sluggish when you feel low or when you aren't sleeping well. A good start to using the workbooks is to do something physical first. For example, get up and walk around the room and – if you have them – up and down the stairs. Then sit down in a chair like a kitchen chair that is upright and forces you to sit straight rather than slump back. Now start reading the workbook. Have some pens and paper handy so you can make notes and write in the book.

If you feel tired halfway through, stop, get physically going again, stretch, have some cold water, then get back to it.

But my life is too busy/unpredictable to use the course

Wouldn't it be great if we could always just sit down and plan a time to work? But sometimes life is busy, unpredictable or hard. If so, just take the time you can.

Here are some suggestions of how to build on this first step during the rest of the course.

Some dos and don'ts for getting the most out of the course

Do:

- Slow it down. Focus on using and applying just one workbook at a time.

- **Get a pen**. Writing things down means you are thinking and learning. In fact it's more than that. Sometimes **you actually work out what you really think** about something when you write it down.

  - Write it down. Things can look different when we write them down. We can notice patterns and habits we might otherwise miss. Sometimes we can start to really work out what is happening when we see it on a page in black and white. Therefore, answer the questions straight away rather than thinking you will come back to it later.

  - You might not wish to write in the book – it may be something you don't like to do or you may have borrowed the book from a library or someone else. If so, you can write your answers on a separate sheet of paper.

  - Many of the worksheets in the course are also available for download from www.llttf.com/odlm

- Answer all the questions – and do try to stop, think and reflect as you read.

- Ask: How might I use this in my life?

- Try out what you read in the workbooks. You'll find a *Planner sheet* at the end of each workbook to help you to decide how to do this.

- Be realistic. You are more likely to succeed if you try changing things one step at a time rather than throwing yourself into things and then running out of steam.

- Re-read the workbooks. You may find that different parts become clearer or seem more useful on reading a second time.

- Use the workbooks to build up the help you receive in other ways, such as talking to friends, or from self-help organizations and support groups.

- Keep it organized and easy to handle. Create your own resource pack of key worksheets and other resources you use to improve how you feel.

- Log on to **www.llttf.com** to get access to free modules and resources.

Don't:

- Push and read through the entire workbook in one go. You need time to take it in and time to practice.

- Expect a sudden miracle cure. Change takes time and practice.

- Try to do this completely on your own. Supportive encouragement from a health professional or social care worker can really help you keep on track.

- Try to read the workbook when you are distracted, such as times when you are trying to do other tasks.

- Cut yourself off from other useful supports. You can do this course alongside other treatments, such as seeing your doctor or taking an antidepressant. These approaches can all be helpful parts of moving forward.

Finding extra support

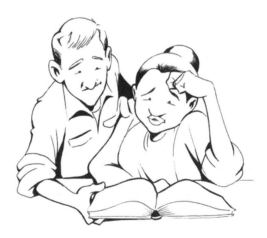

Having someone around who can offer *support and encouragement* can help. This is especially important if you are struggling or feel stuck. Sometimes just the act of telling someone – a family member, friend or health worker – that you are working on something, or plan to do a certain activity on a particular day can really help. Just knowing that someone else may ask you how it's going could help spur you to action. You might go through your answers to the questions in the workbooks with them, or keep your answers private and only discuss some of the course content.

Building your motivation to change

Imagine it is 10 years in the future. You have made important changes in your life and things are much better. Write yourself an **encouraging letter** about why you need to make changes now.

Dear (your name)

Signed:

Me

Change takes time and effort

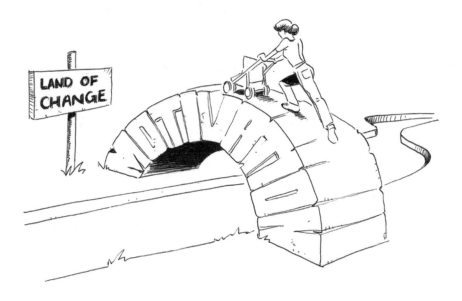

Sometimes it's easy to forget how hard it is to learn new information or skills that you now take for granted. Think about some of the skills you have learned over the years. For example, if you can drive or swim or ride a bike, think back to your first driving/swimming lesson or attempt to cycle without stabilizers. You probably weren't very good at it that first time, yet with practice you developed the skills needed to do it. In the same way, you can help overcome how you feel by practicing what you learn, even if it may seem very hard at first.

Write down some other things you have learned that took time:

> **KEY POINT**
> You can't expect to be able to swim immediately. You may need to start at the shallow end and practice at first. Pace what you do and don't jump straight away into the deep end.

Be realistic

It's important not to approach this course either far too positively or far too negatively. It would be untrue to claim that if you use this course you are guaranteed results. What we can guarantee is that this approach has helped many thousands of people – and that the workbooks teach clinically proved approaches that have been a help for many. Hopefully, at the very least you will learn some interesting and helpful things along the way.

Common problems in using the course

I've no time

Life can be busy and complicated, especially if you have family or work commitments. There will be many demands on your time. But ...

 Task

Imagine you have a close friend who is struggling. They don't like how they feel, and you knew that it is affecting them in lots of different ways. What helpful advice would you give them if they said 'I don't have time'?

Write down your encouraging advice here:

...if you would give your friend advice to make some time, could you use that same advice yourself?

I feel too down to do this now

Sometimes in really severe depression, it might not be the right time to use these workbooks. But you can always come back to them later if you are finding that things are too much now. If you can't concentrate for long just go at a pace you can manage. You should also discuss your treatment options with your doctor.

I'll never change

Perhaps the biggest block to getting better is not believing change can happen. Many people find that they gain much more from the course than they first thought they would. Could this be true for you?

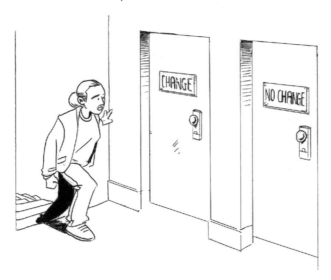

 Task

What words of encouragement would you say to a friend who needed help but believed that change is impossible? Write them down here:

If you would offer helpful and positive advice to a friend, then why not also offer it to yourself?

Experiment

In this course, I'm going to ask you to experiment and try things out. Even if you have doubts about the course, or about your ability to use it effectively, try to give it a go and test out what happens. If you still find it doesn't help at all after you've given it a good go, it would be a sensible time to try something different. But perhaps you'll notice some positive things, even if it's just one or two things. Perhaps that is worth keeping going for.

Summary

Well done – you've got to the last section – and you're still reading! That's a very important achievement. So many people who want to change find it hard starting out.

Let's review what you have learned in this workbook. You have covered:

- How to get the most out of the course.
- How to write a clear but flexible plan of when to use the workbooks.
- How to overcome common blocks to change.

Before you go

 What have I learned from this workbook?

 What do I want to try *next*?

Putting into practice what you have learned

You are likely to make the most progress if you can put into practice what you have learned in the workbook. Each workbook will encourage you to do this by suggesting certain tasks for you to do in the following days.

 Suggested reading

> The *Understanding why you feel as you do* is often a good workbook to read next. It will help you decide which other course workbooks you might need to use.

Making plans

The best plans say:

- **What** you are going to do.

- **When** you are going to do it.

and

- **Predict** things that might block or get in the way of you doing this so you can tackle problems head on.

You may find the following **Planning task** helpful. You can use it to plan any activities or tasks you want – picking a child up from school, getting a repeat prescription, planning to read the next workbook, painting the kitchen – anything.

 Here's an example plan that looks at when and how to start the *Understanding why you feel as you do* workbook. If this is something you would like to do, write your own plan into the Plan below. If you prefer to choose something else, then there are blank versions of this sheet available at the end of the workbook and for download from **www.llttf.com**.

1. What am I going to do?

Suggestion: Start to read the *Why do you feel as you do* workbook

If you decide to do this, think through in more detail exactly what you will do. Do you need to break it down into smaller parts (e.g. get a pen and paper, find the copy of the book or workbook, sit at the table with the door shut and radio off...)? Try to be clear exactly what you will do – so you will be clear when you've done it. Be realistic. Will you plan to read the whole workbook, or just a few pages at a time? Each workbook is also split up into sections that you can work through in smaller sections.

Write what you will do here:

2. When am I going to do it?

What date and time will suit? Many people with low mood notice they feel at their worst first thing in the morning. So you might find that the best time for you to read the workbook is after lunch, in the late afternoon, or in the early evening. If you have young children, think about what you know of their routine. Or you could pick a time when others are around to help look after them. Also, can you plan to read it every day – or do you need a gap to let things sink in?

Write the day and time:

3. Is it well planned?

Next, do a quick reality check on your plan. Is it realistic and well planned? Are you trying to bite off more than you can chew? Is the task small enough for you to succeed, but not so small it makes no difference?

Is my planned task one that:

Q Will be useful for helping me move forward?	Yes ☐	No ☐
Q Is clear, so that I will know when I have done it?	Yes ☐	No ☐
Q Is something that I value, or need to do?	Yes ☐	No ☐
Q Is realistic, practical and achievable?	Yes ☐	No ☐

4. What problems/difficulties could arise, and how can I overcome this?

What could get in the way?

- *Things within you* – low motivation, forgetfulness, talking yourself out of it?
- *Or things outside you* – other people, bad weather, the need for money to do an activity, having to travel or perhaps a task that depends on someone else for success? Unpredictable things may also happen from time to time and interrupt your plans.

Have a back-up time planned for if you can't start working on the course when you first planned. For example, what if a friend unexpectedly drops by for a coffee, or your baby cries, wakes up or needs a nappy change?

Write your possible blocks in here:

Finally, think again about the task and decide whether you need to rewrite your plan to tackle these possible blocks.

5. Write your final plan here:

What are you going to do?

When are you going to do it (day and time)?

During the course, you can make all sorts of future plans using the *Planner sheet* at the end of this workbook. Many people find that by writing things down it helps them organize things and get things sorted.

Plan, Do and Review

Whatever you choose to do, the first step is to make a plan and then do (or not do!) it. The *Planner sheet* will help you create a clear and realistic plan. The next step is to use the *Review sheet* to consider how things have gone, and whether good or bad to learn from it. Copies of both sheets are found at the end of the workbook, and as with all the worksheets can be downloaded from www.llttf.com.

That last part is important. This isn't about having a time for self-congratulation or criticism. It's all about planning effective progress and learning about what works and doesn't in your own life right now.

Look at the *Review sheet*. It asks you to consider whether you completed the planned task or not. If you have managed to do it as planned, then well done. If not, then what stopped you? Was it something inside you like forgetting, or talking yourself out of it? Or was it something outside you like a child being ill, an unexpected accident or friend dropping by, or perhaps it rained? It's all about learning how to plan more effectively. How could you plan things differently the next time to tackle this?

Whichever tasks and workbooks you use on this course, keep coming back to this *Plan, Do, Review* approach. You can even use it to plan the weekly shop!

Other sources of support

 www.llttf.com

This popular resource is designed to support readers of this course and is free to use. There's also a forum where you can make comments, or ask questions of other people who are using the same course.

 www.lttf.com/shop

Access a wide range of Five Areas resources, including free hand-outs and relaxation MP3 files.

Worksheets to help you practice

Practice is important to help you master this approach. You can download worksheets of all the key skills used in this workbook from www.lttf.com/worksheets/odlm

Other resources

Here are details of some other Five Areas resources that can be helpful at times of low or anxious mood.

- *24 hours to get a job that really fires you up.* (Highly Commended BMA book awards) (Kindle)

- *Overcoming anxiety: A Five Areas approach.*

- *Are you strong enough to keep your temper?* (Kindle)

- *I'm not good enough* (low confidence). (Kindle)

- *Stop smoking in 5 minutes.* (Kindle)

- *I feel so bad I can't go on.* (Winner, BMA book awards) (Kindle)

- *Fix your drinking problem in 2 days.* (Kindle) (Linked website: www.llttf4drink.com)

- *Enjoy your baby* (postnatal depression). (Kindle)

- *Reclaim your life from illness, disability, pain or fatigue.* (Kindle)

- *I'm not supposed to feel like this: A Christian self-help approach to depression and anxiety*, C Williams, P Richards and I Whitton (linked website: www.llttfwg.com).

A request for feedback

If there are areas in this course that you find hard to understand, don't work well for you or seemed poorly written, please let me know. I'm sorry I can't answer specific questions or provide advice on treatment.

Email: feedback@fiveareas.com

Address: Five Areas, PO Box 9, Glasgow G63 0WL, UK

In your feedback, please state which workbook, book or website you are commenting on.

Acknowledgments

The cartoon illustrations were produced by Keith Chan, kchan75@hotmail.com. The terms LLTTF and Five Areas are registered trademarks of Five Areas Resources Ltd.

Although we hope you find this book helpful, it's not intended to be a direct substitute for consultative advice with a healthcare professional, nor do we give any assurance about its effectiveness in a particular case. Accordingly, neither the publisher nor the author shall be held liable for any loss or damages arising from its use.

Planner sheet

1. *What* am I going to do?

2. *When* am I going to do it?

Write in the day and time:

3. Is my planned task one that:

Q Will be useful for helping me move forward?   Yes ☐   No ☐

Q Is clear, so that I will know when I have done it?   Yes ☐   No ☐

Q Is something that I value, or need to do?   Yes ☐   No ☐

Q Is realistic, practical and achievable?   Yes ☐   No ☐

4. What problems/difficulties could arise, and how can I overcome this?

What could get in the way? Write your possible blocks in here:

Do you need to rewrite your plan to tackle these possible blocks?

5. Write down your final plan here

What are you going to do?

When are you going to do it? (day and time)

Your back-up plan: Think of another back-up solution you could turn to if for whatever reason there are problems with your plan.

KEY POINT
If you feel worse with symptoms you can still choose to do the planned activity anyway – because it's important.

Review sheet

What did you plan to do?

Write it here.

What happened? Did you attempt the task?   Yes ☐   No ☐

If yes:

● What went well?

● What didn't go so well?

● What have you learned about from what happened?

● How are you going to apply what you've learned?

If not:
What stopped you?

● *Internal factors* (e.g. forgot, not enough time, put it off, concerns I couldn't do it, I couldn't see the point of it, etc.).

● *External factors* (events that happened, work/home issues, etc.).

● How could you have planned to tackle these blocks?

Use the *Plan, Do, Review* approach to help you move forward.

My notes

Understanding why you feel as you do

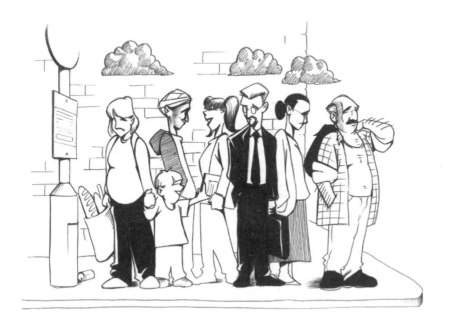

www.llttf.com or www.livinglifetothefull.com 🅱 @llttfnews (public)

www.fiveareas.com 🅱 @fiveareas (practitioners)

📘 www.llttf.com/facebook

Dr Chris Williams

overcoming
depression and low mood
a five areas approach

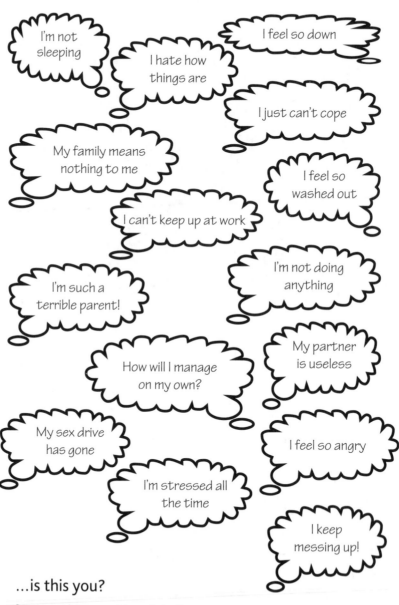

...is this you?

If it is... this workbook is for you.

This workbook will help you to:

- Find out how feelings of low mood, stress and upset are affecting you.
- Choose targets for change that will help you feel better.

Feeling out of balance – when things feel worse and worse

The first step to feeling good is working out why you are feeling bad. Anyone can feel depressed and stressed if their emotional balance is upset.

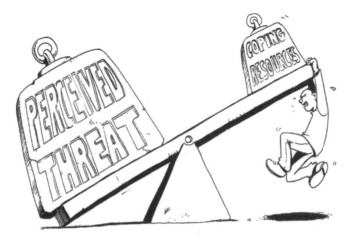

Normally, most people feel **able to cope** with the problems they face. When you are in balance, you know you can deal with your problems. So it isn't your situation or problem alone that causes you to feel down or stressed. Instead it's how you think about these things that makes you feel like you do. And dwelling on problems and getting things out of perspective doesn't help you feel better or make your problem go away.

Q Do I feel in balance at the moment?

Yes ☐   No ☐   Sometimes ☐

If you feel out of balance some or all of the time, this course can help you get your balance back.

Understanding how you feel using the Five Areas approach

Let's start by finding out more about how your lowered mood affects five key areas of your life.

The Five Areas are:

- Area 1: The situations, relationships and practical problems you face. This includes the **people and events** around you.

- Area 2: Your **thinking**. This can often become extreme and unhelpful when you feel distressed.

- Area 3: Your **feelings** (also called moods or emotions).

- Area 4: Any **altered physical symptoms** in your body.

- Area 5: Your **altered behaviour or activity levels**. This includes both the helpful things you can do to make you feel better, and the unhelpful things you do, which backfire and make you feel even worse.

Try to think about how the Five Areas™ assessment can help Paul understand how he is feeling.

Example: How depression is affecting Paul's life

Paul started feeling depressed and was struggling at work. He felt more and more tired. He found it hard to sleep or even relax – even when he went on holiday. He was exhausted and tearful over things he would normally cope with.

By this time, Paul felt he was failing in everything. He was struggling to cope, couldn't sleep and was lying awake, beating himself up that he was feeling like this. He also felt he was letting his partner Helen down. They had many arguments and often lay in bed not speaking. Two months later Paul went off work sick, and eight weeks on he still can't cope with returning to work. He sits at home dwelling on thoughts that he will be laid off. He is doing less and less and stays in all the time. Because he is off work, money worries are also beginning to mount up. This makes him feel even more guilty as he thinks he should be working and bringing in a full wage.

The figure below shows how Paul's problems can be summarized using the Five Areas approach.

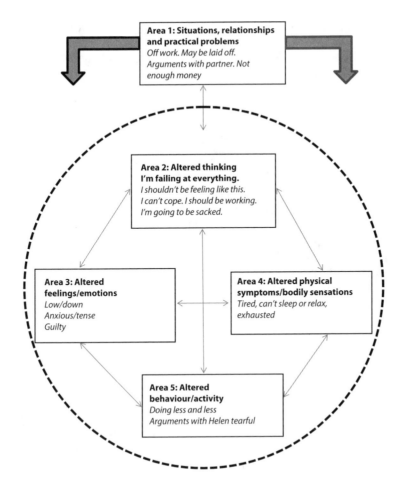

The Five Areas diagram also shows that what you think about a situation or problem can affect how you feel physically and emotionally. It also shows that your thinking affects what you do (your behaviour or activity levels). Look at the arrows in the diagram. Each of the Five Areas of your life affects each other.

 Task

Can the Five Areas approach help you understand why you feel as you do? Take a look at what's happening for you in each of the Five Areas, starting with Area 1.

Area 1: Situations, relationships and practical problems

All of us from time to time face problems such as:

- Problems with family and life at home.
- The challenges of bringing up young children.

- Problems in relationships with partners, neighbours, or friends or colleagues.

- Other life challenges, for example problems at work, college, etc.

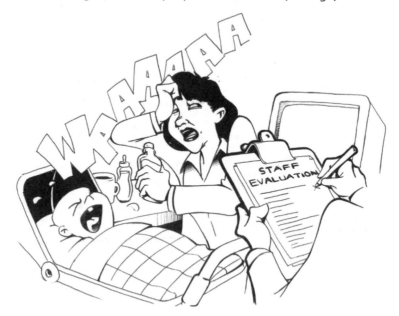

Low mood and tension can affect any kind of relationship. You may become confused about your feelings toward others, and you can lose interest in your relationships. Love can feel subdued. For example, Paul's depression was affecting his feelings for Helen. Similarly, those with a spiritual faith may feel they struggle to get the support that they usually get from their faith.

Are any of these relevant to you?

Situations, relationship or practical problem	*Do you ever face these problems? (Put a tick in the box if these problems are present in your life – even if just sometimes.)* *Write down an example*
1. There is no one around that I can really talk to	
2. I am struggling to cope with my work	
3. I worry about work or money or debts	
4. There are problems where I live/housing problems	
5. It's hard to get on with another person or people in my family	
6. I am having problems with my neighbours	

Situations, relationship or practical problem	Do you ever face these problems? (Put a tick in the box if these problems are present in your life – even if just sometimes.) Write down an example
7. I have problems with colleagues at work	
8. My family has unemployment/job worries	
9. My family has housing problems	
10. My baby isn't feeding/sleeping	
11. My children won't do what I tell them|	

 Task

Now write down any other problems you may have. Use an extra sheet of paper if you need to.

Summary for Area 1: Situations, relationships and practical problems

After answering the questions, rate the extent of your problems in this area.

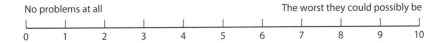

No problems at all   The worst they could possibly be

0   1   2   3   4   5   6   7   8   9   10

Area 2: Your thinking

When someone feels low, how they **think** tends to change. You tend to lose confidence and find it harder to make decisions. You may worry about things you have done – and things you haven't done. You begin to see everything in quite negative ways and fall into negative habits of thinking.

So your thinking becomes:

● Extreme and unhelpful.

Example: How you think can affect how you feel

You are shopping in a supermarket when your 12-month-old daughter starts crying. Nothing you do helps. You give her a cuddle and try to distract her, but she continues to shout and cry. As other shoppers go by you think 'She's doing this on purpose to embarrass me'. You blush and cringe with embarrassment and your body feels very tense. You start to feel really angry and shout at her to 'just shut up and stop whining!' You leave the shop and feel very embarrassed.

But if the same situation occurred and you had thought, 'She must be hungry', you would have felt and behaved differently.

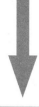

KEY POINT

We can all fall into unhelpful patterns of thinking when we feel low or distressed.

 Have you noticed any of these seven common unhelpful patterns of thinking in your life?

Unhelpful thinking pattern	Do you ever think this way? (Put a tick in the box if you have noticed this thinking style – even if just sometimes.) Write down an example.
1. *Being your own worst critic/bias against yourself* Being very self-critical overlooking your strengths, or not recognizing your achievements	
2. *Putting a negative slant on things* (negative mental filter) Seeing things through dark-tinted glasses; seeing the glass as being half empty rather than half full; that whatever you do in the week it's never enough; focusing on the bad side of everyday situations	
3. *Have a gloomy view of the future* Thinking that things will stay bad or get even worse; predicting that things will go wrong; or always looking for the next thing to fail	
4. *Jumping to the worst conclusion* Predicting that the very worst outcome will happen, thinking that you will fail very badly	

Unhelpful thinking pattern	Do you ever think this way? (Put a tick in the box if you have noticed this thinking style – even if just sometimes.) Write down an example.
5. *Having a negative view about how others see you* (mind-reading) Often thinking that others don't like you or think badly of you for no particular reason	
6. *Unfairly taking responsibility for things* Thinking you should take the blame if things go wrong; feeling guilty about things that are not really your fault; and believing that you are responsible for everyone else	
7. *Making extreme statements/rules* Using the words *'always', 'never'* a lot to summarize things; If a bad thing happens, saying *'Just typical'* because it seems this always happens; Making yourself a lot of *'must', 'should', 'ought'* or *'got to'* rules	

Summary for Area 2: Your thinking

Having answered the questions, rate the extent of your problems in this area.

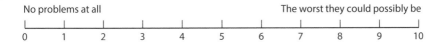

No problems at all   The worst they could possibly be

0   1   2   3   4   5   6   7   8   9   10

Area 3: Your feelings/emotions

What emotional changes have you noticed over the past two weeks?	Put a tick in the box if you are affected by these emotions – even if just sometimes. Write down an example.
Lowness or sadness	
Reduced or no sense of pleasure in things	
Loss of all feelings, for example, noticing no feelings at all	
Guilt	
Worry, stress, tension, anxiety or panic	
Anger or irritability	
Shame or embarrassment	
Other (write down here):	

Summary for Area 3: Your feelings/emotions

Having answered the questions, rate the extent of your problems.

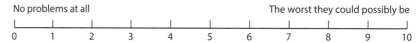

Area 4: Altered physical symptoms

Usually when people feel very low it affects how they feel physically as well.

 Which physical symptoms have you noticed over the past two weeks?

Which altered physical sensations have you noticed?	Put a tick in the box if you have noticed these sensations – even if just sometimes. Write down an example.
Are you waking up earlier than usual?	
Are you finding it hard getting off to sleep?	
Are you waking up at night?	
Has your appetite increased or decreased?	
Have you put on or lost weight?	
Do you feel as if you don't have enough energy to do things?	
If this affects you, have you stopped having sex or aren't interested as much in it as before?	
Are you constipated?	
Do you feel any pain?	
Do you feel restless?	
Do you have any other physical symptoms or problems such as physical illness?	

Summary for Area 4: Altered physical symptoms

Having answered the questions, rate the extent of your problems in this graph.

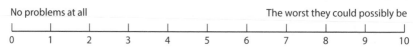

Area 5: Altered behaviour or activity levels

You have already worked hard in thinking about the first four of the five areas in your Five Areas Assessment – well done! Here you look at the last area – altered behaviour (things that you can do).

Many ways in which you respond can be very helpful and boost how you are feeling. However, some things we do can worsen how we feel, such as:

- *Reducing your activity levels* by not doing as much as before.

- *Avoiding or escaping* from doing things that seem scary or too difficult.

- Starting to *respond in ways that backfire* and make you feel worse. For example by pushing others away, losing your temper at others for no good reason or having too much alcohol to block how you feel.

KEY POINT

Making changes in your behaviour and activity levels are some of the most helpful things you can do first to boost how you feel.

A. First type of altered behaviour: Reduced activity

When you feel down, it's hard to keep doing things because you have:

- Low energy and feel tired ('I'm too tired').

- Little sense of enjoyment or achievement when you do things.

- Negative thoughts about things ('I just can't be bothered').

- Everything can seem just too much, so it feels such a relief to do less.

All these lead to reduced activity – where you do less of or stop doing things which are important to you. Often the first things that are squeezed out are things that have previously given you a sense of **fun** or **achievement** (for example, meeting up with friends, and doing things with your family). You can also lose your sense of **closeness** to others.

But the less you do, the worse you feel, and the worse you feel, the less you do – so a vicious circle is set up.

Write down any examples of reduced activity you do here:

The good news is that once you have noticed whether this is true for you, you can start to get going again and that by increasing activity levels, you will start to feel better.

B. Second type of altered behaviour: Avoiding or escaping from things

We often start to avoid or escape from people, places and situations that make us anxious. This may make you feel better in the short term and this explains why it's so easy to get into cycles of doing less and less. But in the longer term, avoiding things makes it harder and harder to confidently face your fears in the future. And you don't see that your worst fears don't actually occur. In fact, avoidance teaches us the unhelpful rule that we only coped with a situation by avoiding it.

KEY POINT
Avoidance and escaping can make you feel worse and also undermine your confidence.

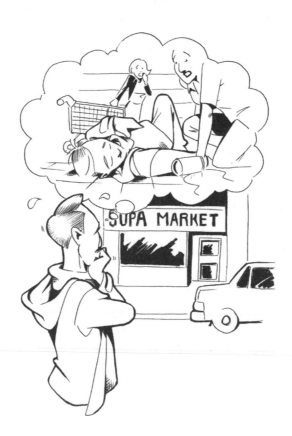

Write down any examples of avoidance you do here:

> **KEY POINT**
> The good news is that once you have noticed if this is true for you, you can start working on tackling avoidance and facing your fears.

C. Third type of altered behaviour: Dropping helpful responses

Helpful behaviours include doing things such as:

- Talking to friends or family for support.

- Going to see a doctor or healthcare practitioner to discuss whether you need extra help.

- Finding activities or meeting people that give you a boost.

- If you have a personal spiritual faith, your beliefs may provide helpful support.

Write down any examples of helpful behaviours you do here:

D. Fourth type of altered behaviour: Unhelpful things you do

Sometimes people may do things that make them feel better at first but in the longer term backfire and make them feel worse. Do you do any of the following unhelpful behaviours?

- Withdrawing into yourself and cutting yourself off from your friends or family.

- Neglecting yourself (for example, by not eating as much or not washing).

- Doing things that clash with your values/ideals and you really know are not how you want to live. This might include deliberately taking risks, picking fights or betraying a partner.

- Being rude and critical, or pushing people away to see how much they really want to support you.

- Drinking excessively, or using street drugs to block how you feel.

● Harming yourself as a way of blocking how you feel.

Write down any examples of unhelpful behaviour you do here:

You can find out more about reducing unhelpful behaviours in the workbook *Unhelpful things you do*.

Summary for Area 5: Any altered behaviours/activity levels

Now think about all the altered behaviours you have identified and rate the extent of your problems in this area.

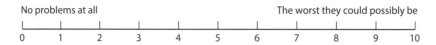

No problems at all   The worst they could possibly be

0   1   2   3   4   5   6   7   8   9   10

What next?

Remember that the purpose of the Five Areas approach is to help you work out how your low mood is affecting you. It can help you plan the areas you need to focus on to bring about change.

The good news is that all the areas are linked so that making changes in any one area can lead to change in the others. So if you try to alter any one of these areas by working through a workbook in the course, it will help lift your low mood and help you tackle feeling low or stressed.

Where do you start?

KEY POINT

One key to success is to try not to tackle everything at once. You are more likely to improve if you take slow steady steps than if you are too enthusiastic at the start and then run out of steam. So try to take things one step at a time by choosing the areas you are going to focus on to start with.

Set yourself:

● *Short-term targets*: these are changes you can make today, tomorrow and next week.

● *Medium-term targets*: these are changes to be put in place over the next few weeks.

● *Long-term targets*: this is where you want to be in six months or a year.

Overcoming Anxiety, Stress and Panic © Dr Chris Williams 2015

Which workbook should you try first?

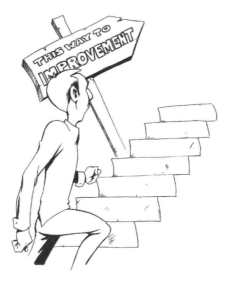

Your Five Areas assessment will help you choose which workbooks to read first. Pick just one area and one workbook of the course first. This means that you are actively choosing not to focus on the other areas to start with. Choose something that will make a difference now. Because each of the five areas affects each other, choosing any of the areas to start on makes sense. Just choose something **you** want to work on.

If you want help in deciding where to start, we recommend you read the workbooks in this order:

- The *Doing things that boost how you feel* workbook can help you quickly re-set a pattern to your day, and plan activities that will make you feel better soon.

- If you are sleeping poorly, use the *Overcoming sleep problems* workbook.

- If you are taking or thinking of taking an antidepressant try reading *Understanding and using antidepressant medication* as soon as you can.

If you have a close family member or friend you'd like to help you in using the course, ask them to read the *Information for families and friends* workbook. You also may find it helpful.

Please note: there is no such thing as a set 'course' in this book. The course is as many or as few workbooks as you feel you need to use.

Tick which workbooks you want to read in the table below. Place a * by the first workbook you intend to work on.

Workbook	Plan to read	Tick when completed
Starting out – and how to keep going if you feel stuck		
Understanding why you feel as you do		
Making changes to do with people and events		
Practical problem solving		
Being assertive		
Building relationships with your family and friends		
Information for families and friends – how can you offer the best support?		
Making changes to behaviours and activity levels		
Doing things that boost how you feel		
Using exercise to boost how you feel		
Helpful things you can do		
Unhelpful things you do		
Making changes to negative and upsetting thinking		
Noticing and changing extreme and unhelpful thinking		
Changing extreme and unhelpful thinking		
Making changes to things that affect your bodily well-being		
Overcoming sleep problems		
Alcohol, drugs and you		
Understanding and using antidepressant medication		
Making changes for the future		
Planning for the future		

KEY POINT
Repeat your **Five Areas assessment** after using each workbook to help you decide where to go next.

Overcoming Anxiety, Stress and Panic © Dr Chris Williams 2015

How do I know if I need extra help?

Ideally anyone using these workbooks will have someone to support them in doing it. But there are times when this won't be enough. If you struggle to do the tasks in the workbooks don't worry. Just do what you can. But if things *still* do not seem to be improving, you may need to get extra help.

If you have somebody supporting you, discuss what you have been doing with them. Otherwise make an appointment to see your doctor or a mental health worker.

You *really need* to get extra help for:

- **Severe depression**, for example, continuing low mood, tearfulness, not eating or drinking much at all or a big loss of weight, despite attempts to improve things.

- Strong urges to **self-harm** or feeling really **hopeless or suicidal** about the future.

- Strong urges to harm anyone else.

- Other **dangerous behaviours**, for example, risk-taking, threats of harm to others.

- Not being able to cope so much that you are concerned about the health and well-being of those around you, such as your child or children.

- Severe withdrawal from life activities.

KEY POINT
It is better to ask for help or advice than do nothing.

Getting extra help

You can ask:

- **Someone you can trust** – or you may find it easier to talk to someone outside your closest friends and family. Don't feel guilty if this is the case, it's actually normal to feel like this.

- **Your doctor**. He or she can give you medical advice and (if he or she feels it is necessary) refer you to a specialist mental health worker or team for a fuller assessment.

- **Social services**. Social workers can be a great source of support. Look in your local directory or online for your local office's number and a 24-hour emergency number for initial referrals and queries.

Other organizations/sources you can approach for help are listed on the **www.llttf .com** website.

Summary

In this workbook you have:

- Understood what is low mood and depression.
- Learned how to complete your own Five Areas assessment to check how you are feeling.
- Discovered how to choose which other course workbooks you should use.
- Learned when you should get extra help and where to go for it.

Before you go

 What have I learned from this workbook?

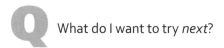 What do I want to try *next*?

Putting into practice what you have learned

You are likely to make the most progress if you can put into practice what you have learned in the workbook. Each workbook will encourage you to do this by suggesting certain tasks for you to do in the following days.

 Task

At the end of each day, complete a blank Five Areas assessment sheet (available at the end of this workbook). More copies are available for download at **www .llttf.com**.

Choose a time when you have felt better, and a time when you have felt worse, and complete the sheets.

Plan, Do and Review

Whatever you choose to do, the first step is to make a plan and then do (or not do!) it. The *Planner sheet* will help you create a clear and realistic plan. The next step is to use the *Review sheet* to consider how things have gone, and whether good or bad to learn from it. Copies of both sheets are found at the end of the workbook, and as with all the worksheets can be downloaded from www.llttf.com.

Other sources of support

 www.llttf.com (www.livinglifetothefull.com; 🅑 @llttfnews)

This popular resource is designed to support readers of this course. There's also a forum where you can make comments, or ask questions of other people using the same course.

Acknowledgments

The cartoon illustrations were produced by Keith Chan, kchan75@hotmail.com.

The terms LLTTF and Five Areas are registered trademarks of Five Areas Resources Ltd.

Although we hope you find this book helpful, it's not intended to be a direct substitute for consultative advice with a healthcare professional, nor do we give any assurance about its effectiveness in a particular case. Accordingly, neither the publisher nor the author shall be held liable for any loss or damages arising from its use.

Use this worksheet to note down how your current situation, thoughts, feelings, physical symptoms and behaviour may be affecting your life. You can then begin to identify ways to change things in ways that could enhance your daily life.

Your Five Areas Assessment

Situation, relationships and practical problems

Altered thinking

Altered feelings/emotions

Altered physical symptoms

Altered behaviour/activity levels

Overcoming Anxiety, Stress and Panic © Dr Chris Williams 2015

Planner sheet

1. *What* am I going to do?

2. *When* am I going to do it?

Write in the day and time:

3. Is my planned task one that:

Will be useful for helping me move forward?	Yes ☐	No ☐
Is clear, so that I will know when I have done it?	Yes ☐	No ☐
Is something that I value, or need to do?	Yes ☐	No ☐
Is realistic, practical and achievable?	Yes ☐	No ☐

4. What problems/difficulties could arise, and how can I overcome this?

What could get in the way? Write your possible blocks in here:

Do you need to rewrite your plan to tackle these possible blocks?

5. Write down your final plan here.

What are you going to do?

When are you going to do it? (day and time)

Your back-up plan: Think of another back-up solution you could turn to if for whatever reason there are problems with your plan.

KEY POINT
If you feel worse with symptoms you can still choose to do the planned activity anyway – because it's important.

Review sheet

What did you plan to do?

Write it here.

What happened? Did you attempt the task?   Yes ☐   No ☐

If yes:

● What went well?

● What didn't go so well?

● What have you learned about from what happened?

● How are you going to apply what you've learned?

If not:

What stopped you?

● *Internal factors* (e.g. forgot, not enough time, put it off, concerns I couldn't do it, I couldn't see the point of it, etc.)

● *External factors* (events that happened, work/home issues, etc.)

● How could you have planned to tackle these blocks?

Use the *Plan, Do, Review* approach to help you move forward.

Worksheets to help you practice *Understanding why you feel as you do*

Practice is important to help you master this approach. You can download worksheets of all of the key skills used in this workbook from:
www.llttf.com/worksheets/odlm

My notes

Part 2
Making changes

Practical problem solving

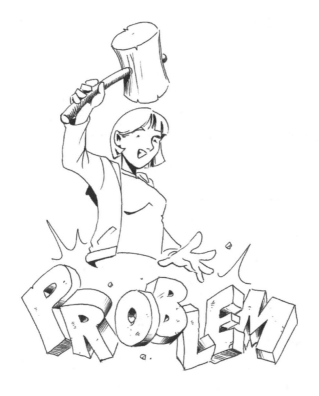

www.llttf.com or www.livinglifetothefull.com 🇪 @llttfnews (public)

www.fiveareas.com 🇪 @fiveareas (practitioners)

www.llttf.com/facebook

Dr Chris Williams

overcoming
depression and low mood
a five areas approach

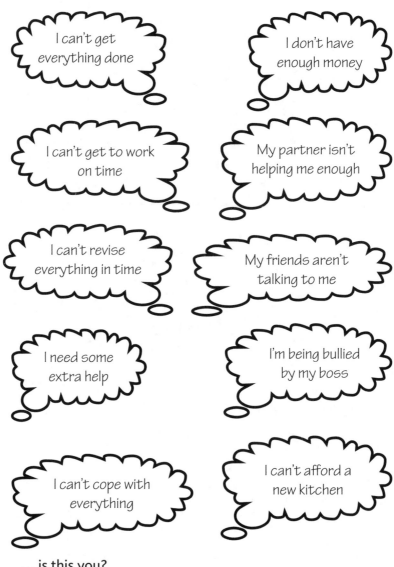

... is this you?
If so... this workbook is for you.

     Overcoming Anxiety, Stress and Panic © Dr Chris Williams 2015

In this workbook you will:

- Learn how practical problems can affect life.
- Identify practical problems in your own life.
- See an example of problem solving in practice and apply it to a problem of your own.

How practical problems affect us

Everyone faces some problems and difficulties in life. This workbook focuses on practical problems that go on outside us – difficult situations, other people and practical difficulties that we all face from time to time. Often, you can cope when there's just one problem. But when you face a particularly hard problem or a whole lot of smaller things all at the same time, you can struggle to cope and feel overwhelmed. This is especially so when you're feeling tired or ground down.

Think back to the Five Areas assessment you completed in the *Understanding why you feel as you do* workbook. The first of the five areas is the situations, relationships and practical problems we face. These problems don't just stay outside us – they affect us inside as well. They can affect what we think about (altered thinking, area 2), how we feel emotionally (altered feelings, area 3) and how we react in our bodies (altered physical symptoms/bodily sensations, area 4), and finally all add up to affect what we do (area 5, our altered behaviour or activity levels).

By making changes in any of these areas, there can be positive changes in each of the others. Tackling these problems will therefore help you feel better, and this workbook will help you achieve this.

Before you start

Sometimes problems occur because of things we can't control. But sometimes they're the result of things that could have been done differently. For example, problems in relationships may build up because one person ignored a misunderstanding and kept expecting the other person to do something but without making it clear what was needed.

- Or, perhaps they didn't respond in ways that would have prevented things worsening at an earlier stage ("*a stitch in time*....").

- Or maybe a problem of debt has built up because of problem gambling or drinking?

Therefore, before you start working on the plan you need to think about these three things:

1. **Your behaviour:** Do you find that the same kinds of problems occur again and again? If so, is there anything that you keep doing (or not doing) that leads to the problem? If you answered 'Yes', you may find the workbook on *Unhelpful things you do* useful.

2. **Your thinking:** Is it possible that things are being blown up out of all proportion because of how you feel inside at the moment? If you think this may be so, then try reading the *Noticing* and the *Changing extreme and unhelpful thinking* workbooks to help you get things back into perspective.

3. **Other people and other ways of support:** Some problems are hard to change by yourself. So check out who is there around you whom you could ask to support you if you feel you can't do this on your own.

 Task

Make a list of any practical resources and supports that you have.

At times of distress, people sometimes seem aware of only the problems. You may overlook or downplay your strengths. This can make you ignore the supports you have just listed above even though they are there. Remember: the supports you have listed may be part of your solution.

How to tackle problems

- Approach each problem separately, and in turn.

- Define the problem clearly so that you are focused in your work.

But what if the problem seems really huge or seems really complicated? Well, when problems are large like that, it's a bit like facing the challenge of how would you eat an elephant.

How do you eat an elephant – or if you are vegetarian, a huge turnip? Of course, you'd eat it one bit at a time. In the same way, you can break down any problem – no matter how large or complicated, into smaller parts that are then easier to solve.

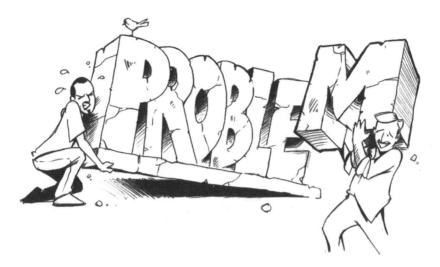

Have a clear plan

You will need to decide:

- **Short-term** targets – changes you can make today, tomorrow and next week.

- **Medium-term** targets – changes over the next few weeks.

- **Long-term** targets – where you want to be in six months or a year.

That way you can tackle even very big or complicated problems step by step.

The seven steps to problem solving

Step 1: Identify and clearly define what you are going to work on

Below is a list of common difficult situations, practical and relationship problems. Are any of these affecting you? Most people face many issues every day, so it's likely that you will have noticed problems in at least some of these areas. You can also add any other problems to the space at the end of the table.

Difficult situations, relationships and practical issues	Yes	No	Sometimes
I have worries about money or debts	☐	☐	☐
There are problems where I live	☐	☐	☐
I/somebody close to me doesn't have a job	☐	☐	☐

(Continued)

	Yes	No	Sometimes
I/somebody close to me doesn't enjoy their job	☐	☐	☐
I don't have time to do everything needed around the house	☐	☐	☐
I don't have time to do everything needed in my other commitments outside the house/family	☐	☐	☐
There's something I need to buy or borrow	☐	☐	☐
There's too much to do in the available time	☐	☐	☐
There's something practical I don't understand that I need to find out about	☐	☐	☐
There's an item that's broken/damaged/leaking that needs fixing	☐	☐	☐
Relationship issues	*Yes*	*No*	*Sometimes*
There is no-one around whom I can really talk to	☐	☐	☐
I have relationship issues (such as arguments) with my partner/spouse	☐	☐	☐
My partner/spouse doesn't really talk to me or offer me enough support	☐	☐	☐
I have relationship issues (such as arguments) with close family members, for example, parents/brother/sister	☐	☐	☐
I'm not spending time with my children like I want to	☐	☐	☐
My children won't do what I tell them	☐	☐	☐
Someone close to me has alcohol or drug problems	☐	☐	☐
Someone close to me has problems with the police or courts	☐	☐	☐
Someone close to me is being threatened by somebody	☐	☐	☐
There's someone else, like a sick relative, I have to care for	☐	☐	☐
I have difficulties with others, for example, neighbours/friends/colleagues at work	☐	☐	☐

Write down any other difficult situations, relationship or practical issues you are facing here (remember these are problems outside you):

 Example: Julia's practical problem

Julia's son Ben is 11 years old and is going to start high school in September. He needs a new uniform, but Julia doesn't have enough money. She ticks several boxes in the list of problems above, and decides the one she wants to focus on is: *There's something I need to buy or borrow – the uniform.*

Now it's your turn

Look back at your responses and choose **one** problem that you will tackle first. This is particularly important if you have ticked many boxes in the list. It isn't possible to overcome all these problems at once, so you need to decide which **one** area to focus on.

My target problem: Write down the one problem area you want to work on first.

 KEY POINT
Remember that this should be a practical or relationship problem.

Break it into smaller steps if you need to.

Breaking it down into smaller steps

The important thing is to use a **step-by-step** approach where no single step seems too large. And the first step needs to be something that gets you moving in the right direction.

 Example: Julia's step-by-step

Julia decides to break down the task – getting the new uniform – into some smaller steps. This is because she doesn't have enough money to just go out and buy it. She therefore decides that as a first step she will **try to buy a second-hand uniform**.

Now decide whether you need to break your target into smaller steps.

Is it a big and difficult task like eating an elephant? Do you need to break it down into smaller, more achievable steps that you can tackle over the next week or two?

Yes ☐   No ☐

If you answered 'No', then please go straight to Step 2. If you answered 'Yes', then what smaller steps could help you move forward? If you need to, write down your revised first target here again:

Step 2: Think up as many solutions as possible to achieve your first target

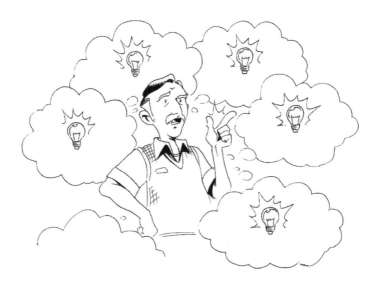

When you feel overwhelmed by practical problems, often it's hard to see a way out. It can seem hard to even start tackling the problem.

One way around this is to step back from the problem and see if any other solutions are possible. This approach is called **brainstorming**. The more solutions that you can think of, the more likely it is that a good one will emerge.

The purpose of brainstorming is to try to come up with **as many ideas as possible**. And then it will be easier for you to identify a good solution.

KEY POINT
You can even include ridiculous ideas at first as you are just trying to get yourself to start thinking more flexibly!

Think:

Q What advice would you give a friend who was trying to make the same changes? Sometimes it's easier to think of solutions for others than for ourselves.

Q What *ridiculous* solutions can you include as well as more sensible ones?

Q What helpful ideas would others (e.g. family, friends or colleagues) suggest?

Q What have you tried in the past that was helpful before?

Example: Julia's problem – possible solutions

(Including ridiculous ideas at first)

- Ignore the problem completely – he can make do with what he has.
- I could steal some clothes from someone's washing line.
- I could see if the uniform is available second-hand on the Internet.
- I can look in the local paper/free sheet and see if there's anything available.
- I could ask round my friends and relatives and see if they have one/any ideas.
- I could put a 'Wanted' card up at the newsagent.

Now write down as many possible solutions (including ridiculous ideas at first) for your own problem:

Step 3: Look at the pros and cons of each possible solution

 Example: Julia writes down the pros and cons of her solutions

Suggestion	Pros (advantages)	Cons (disadvantages)
Ignore the problem completely – he can make do with what he has	Easier in the short term and I don't have to think about it. He can manage without it for the start of term	Well, Ben's growing and won't fit the clothes he now has and there is a strict dress code – we'll need to get the uniform soon
I could steal the clothes from someone's washing line	Well it might work, but...	I don't want to do that – it's wrong. It's one of my whacky brainstorm ideas. Even if I did think like that I wouldn't. I'd get fined and have even less money than I have now
I could see if the uniform is available second-hand on the Internet	That's a good idea – people often advertise lots of stuff at a good price	There might not be one for sale there. What's the chance of finding our local school's uniform there?
I can look in the local paper/free sheet and see if there's anything available	That's another good idea – they have loads of pages with local stuff for sale and may include school uniform!	I'd need to spend time looking through the pages and then follow it up
I could ask round my friends and relatives and see if they have one/any ideas	Lots of them have had children. One of them may well have a uniform they want to get rid of	I'd have to spend time getting in touch with them all
I could put a 'Wanted' card up at the newsagent	Well, I've seen other people do this. It must work sometimes	I'd feel a bit nervous asking the newsagent if I could put it up. Do you have to pay for that sort of thing?

Write **your own** list of ideas below, and the pros and cons of each suggestion.

My suggestions from Step 2	Pros (advantages)	Cons (disadvantages)

Step 4: Now choose one of the solutions

In making your decision, bear in mind that the best way of tackling a problem is to plan **steady, slow changes**.

KEY POINT

The solution you are looking for is something that gets you moving in the right direction. This should be small enough to be possible, but big enough to move you forward.

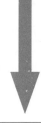

Example: Julia's final choice

Julia tries to choose an option that will make a sensible first step in achieving her goal. She knows her chosen solution should be realistic and then it will be likely to succeed. She makes her decision after looking at all the pros and cons she's listed in Step 3.

Julia decides on balance to first **ask her friends and relatives**. Many of the other suggestions might also work, but this suggestion seems a reasonable first step.

Look at your own responses in Step 3 and then choose a solution.

My solution:

Write down your preferred option here:

Check your solution:

Now see if you can answer 'Yes' to the questions below.

Is my planned solution one that:

Will be useful for helping me move forward?	Yes ☐	No ☐
Is clear, so that I will know when I have done it?	Yes ☐	No ☐
Is something that I value, or need to do?	Yes ☐	No ☐
Is realistic, practical and achievable?	Yes ☐	No ☐

If you answered 'Yes' to all four questions, your chosen step is a good choice to start with. If you answered 'No', then think again and choose another option from your list.

Step 5: Plan the steps needed to carry out your chosen solution

You need to have a clear plan that lays out exactly **what** you are going to do and **when** you are going to do it. *Write down* the steps needed to carry out your plan. Use the *Planner sheet* at the end of this workbook to help you do this. This will help you to think what to do and also to predict possible problems that might arise. Remember that an important part of the planning process is to predict what would block the plan. That way you can think about how you will respond if there were problems to keep your plan on track.

Example: Julia's plan

Who do I know? None of my sisters' children went to the same school. I need to ask my friends. I think the first person I'll ask is Jamila. She knows absolutely everyone and what's what. She's also really confident, so she'll feel able to ask around. And I'll also ask my other friend Andrea. She works next door to a charity shop and she could have a look out for me.

Now, let's think again. Is that a plan that makes clear what I'm going to do and when I'm going to do it? Yes it is. I'll phone them just now while Ben is out playing football. I don't think this plan will be blocked or prevented by anything – unless someone pops by without warning. If so, I'll remember to phone later.

My back-up plan: If none of my friends can help me within a few days, I can always go back to my brainstorm at Step 2, and put up an advert at the newsagent.

Now, write down your plan.

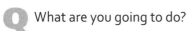 What are you going to do?

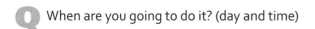 When are you going to do it? (day and time)

Q What problems or difficulties could arise?

Q How could you overcome them?

Choose a back-up plan:

It's good to have a back-up solution for if major difficulties arise with your first choice plan.

 Example: Julia's back-up solution

Julia decides that if her first choice plan doesn't work, she will put an advert in the local newsagent.

Write your own back-up plan here:

Step 6: Carry out your plan

Now carry out your plan during the next week.

Good luck!

Step 7: Review the outcome

Whatever happens, now is the time to review the plan and learn from what happened. Review what happens with the *Review sheet* (copies of which are found later in this workbook).

Now write down your own Review here:

Example 1: Julia's review of a plan that works

What happened? Julia carries out her plan. She phones the people she knows and they promise to help. She thinks she won't hear anything back for a few days, but then Andrea phones back. Andrea was chatting to the person who helps at the local charity shop, and they have got a lot of school-age clothes there. Apparently lots of people have cleared out clothes during the summer. Julia thanks Andrea and as soon as Ben gets home they go to the shop. They manage to get almost all the clothes he needs apart from the sports shoes – and at a good price too. The plan has worked well – leaving just the sports shoes to get.

- *What went well?* It was a good solution.
- *What didn't go so well?* Nothing really.
- *What have you learned about from what happened?* Plans can work well. Friends can be a great resource. It was the right time of year to be looking.
- *How are you going to apply what you have learned?* Next year I could look in the shop at this time of year and may well find things. It might not work at other times of the year though.

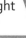

Example 2: Julia's plan doesn't work

- *What happened?* Julia carries out her plan. She phones the people she knows and they all promise to help. But after four days no-one has phoned back.
- *What went well?* I managed to call my friends. They all were friendly and it was nice chatting anyway.
- *What didn't go so well?* It's a shame no-one got back to me.
- *What have you learned about from what happened?* It can seem a good plan but still not work out.
- *How are you going to apply what you've learned?* Julia is disappointed, but she already knows what she will do now (her back-up plan). She will put an advertisement at the newsagent.

She then plans what to do next using a *Planner sheet* at the end of this workbook. She asks Jamila to come to the shop with her for moral support. They find out that Julia can put up the advertisement for free. She puts it on the wall next to the till where people queue. Two days later Julia gets a call from someone who is willing to sell the clothes at a good price.

Q What did you plan to do?

What happened? Did you attempt the task?

Yes ☐   No ☐

If yes:

● What went well?

● What didn't go so well?

● What have you learned about from what happened?

● How are you going to apply what you've learned?

If not:

What stopped you?

● *Internal factors* (e.g. forgot, not enough time, put it off, concerns I couldn't do it, I couldn't see the point of it etc.)

● *External factors* (events that happened, work/home issues, etc.)

● How could you have planned to tackle these blocks?

Use the *Plan, Do, Review* approach to help you move forward.

Overcoming Anxiety, Stress and Panic © Dr Chris Williams 2015

If you noticed problems with your plan

Choosing realistic targets for change is important. Think back to where you started – were you too ambitious or unrealistic in choosing the target you did? Sometimes your attempt to solve a problem may be blocked by something unexpected. Perhaps something didn't happen as you planned, or someone reacted in an unexpected way? Try to learn from what happened.

 How could you change how you approach the problem to help you make a realistic action plan?

Planning the next steps

After completing the first step you need to plan another change to build on this. You will need to slowly build on what you have done in a step-by-step way.

Did your plan help you to tackle the problem you were working on completely? If not, you may need to plan out other solutions to tackle what is left of your problem.

If you are tackling a big or complex problem (like eating an elephant or huge turnip), what is the next bit to chew on?

The important thing is to build one step upon another.

So, you now have the choice to:

- Focus on the same problem area and plan to keep working on it one step at a time.

- Choose a new problem area to work on.

Steps should each always be realistic, practical and achievable. Without a step-by-step approach you may find that although you take some steps forward, these can be all in different directions. So you could lose your focus and motivation. Use what you have just learned to build on what you did.

Consider your **short-term, medium-term** and **longer-term** targets. This means, where you want to be in a few weeks' time (short term), in a few months' time (long term) or in a year's time (long term).

Example: Julia's final choice

Julia has now found all the clothes for Ben apart from the sports shoes. How can she plan to get these?

Julia creates a new seven-step plan. Using the plan, she decides to visit the local shoe warehouse and finds some shoes at a bargain price. She finds a pair that is almost as good value as buying second-hand and she buys them.

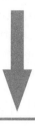

Julia has now sorted out her problem and bought the uniform she wanted for her son. And she could buy at a price she could afford. Now it's your turn.

Your own next steps

When making your next plan:

Do:

- Plan to work on **only** one or two key problems over the next week.

- Plan to alter things slowly in a step-by-step way.

- Use the *Planner sheet* at the end of this workbook to check that each step is always well planned. That way you know exactly what you are going to do and when you'll do it.

Don't:

- Try to start to alter too many things all at once.

- Choose something that is too hard a target to start with.

- Talk yourself out of trying to sort out the problem by saying "*It won't work*" or '*It's a waste of time*'. Try to test out if this negative thinking is actually true by acting against this. Try the plan out and see what happens. You may be pleasantly surprised.

Write your own short-, medium- and long-term plans here:

- **Short term** – What might you do over the next week or so? This is your next step that you need to plan.

- **Medium term** – What might you aim toward doing over the next few weeks – the next few steps?

- **Longer term** – Where do you want to be in a few months or so?

Remember to plan slow, steady changes. By breaking down problems and tackling them one step at a time any problem can be addressed. Use the *Planner sheet* and *Review sheet* to help you get into a system of *Plan, Do and Review*. Copies of both sheets are found at the end of the workbook, and as with all the worksheets can be downloaded from www.llttf.com.

When you need more help

Remember, you are not alone. If you need more help consider asking:

- People around you who you know and trust.

- Your doctor/physician, health visitor or social worker.

- Specialist services and voluntary organizations for help with problems such as debt, housing difficulty and relationship counselling. They can be part of your plan.

A longer list of supports is provided at the **www.llttf.com** website.

Summary

In this workbook you have:

- Learned how practical problems affect your life.
- Learned how to identify problems in your own life that you can change.
- Seen an example of problem solving in practice and applied this to one of your own problems.

Before you go

What have you learned from this workbook?

What do you want to try *next*?

Putting into practice what you have learned

Continue to put into practice what you learn over the next few weeks. Don't try to solve every problem all at once. Plan out what to do at a pace that's right for you. Build changes one step at a time.

 KEY POINT
Don't put off asking for help if you are stuck.

Plan, Do and Review

Whatever you choose to do, the first step is to make a plan and then try it out. The *Planner sheet* will help you create a clear and realistic plan. The next step is to use the *Review sheet* to consider how things have gone, and whether good or bad to learn from it. Copies of both sheets are found at the end of the workbook, and as with all the worksheets can be downloaded from www.llttf.com.

Other sources of support

 www.llttf.com (www.livinglifetothefull.com; @llttfnews)

This popular resource is designed to support readers of this course. There's also a forum where you can make comments, or ask questions of other people using the same course.

Worksheets to help you practice

Practice is important to help you master this approach. You can download worksheets of all the key skills used in this workbook from: www.llttf.com/worksheet /odlm

Acknowledgments

The cartoon illustrations were produced by Keith Chan, kchan75@hotmail.com.

The terms LLTTF and Five Areas are registered trademarks of Five Areas Resources Ltd.

Although we hope you find this book helpful, it's not intended to be a direct substitute for consultative advice with a healthcare professional, nor do we give any assurance about its effectiveness in a particular case. Accordingly, neither the publisher nor the author shall be held liable for any loss or damages arising from its use.

Planner sheet

1. *What* am I going to do?

2. *When* am I going to do it?

Write in the day and time:

3. Is my planned task one that will be:

Q Will be useful for helping me move forward?   Yes ☐   No ☐

Q Is clear, so that I will know when I have done it?   Yes ☐   No ☐

Q Is something that I value, or need to do?   Yes ☐   No ☐

Q Is realistic, practical and achievable?   Yes ☐   No ☐

4. What problems/difficulties could arise, and how can I overcome this?

What could get in the way? Write your possible blocks in here:

Do you need to rewrite your plan to tackle these possible blocks?

5. Write down your final plan here.

What are you going to do?

When are you going to do it? (day and time)

Your back-up plan: Think of another back-up solution you could turn to if for whatever reason there are problems with your plan.

KEY POINT

If you feel worse with symptoms you can still choose to do the planned activity anyway – because it's important.

Overcoming Anxiety, Stress and Panic © Dr Chris Williams 2015

Review sheet

What did you plan to do?

Write it here.

What happened? Did you attempt the task?   Yes ☐   No ☐

If yes:

- What went well?

- What didn't go so well?

- What have you learned about from what happened?

- How are you going to apply what you've learned?

If not:

What stopped you?

- *Internal factors* (e.g. forgot, not enough time, put it off, concerns I couldn't do it, I couldn't see the point of it, etc.).

- *External factors* (events that happened, work/home issues, etc.).

- How could you have planned to tackle these blocks?

Use the *Plan, Do, Review* approach to help you move forward.

Worksheets to help you practice *Practical problem solving*

Practice is important to help you master this approach. You can download worksheets of all of the key skills used in this workbook from:
www.llttf.com/worksheets/odlm

My notes

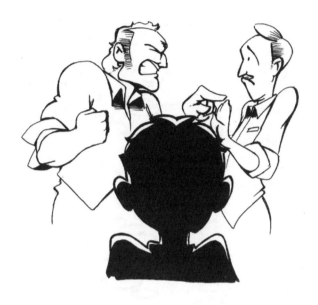

www.llttf.com or www.livinglifetothefull.com 🅱 @llttfnews (public)

www.fiveareas.com 🅱 @fiveareas (practitioners)

🅵www.llttf.com/facebook

Dr Chris Williams

overcoming
depression and low mood
a five areas approach

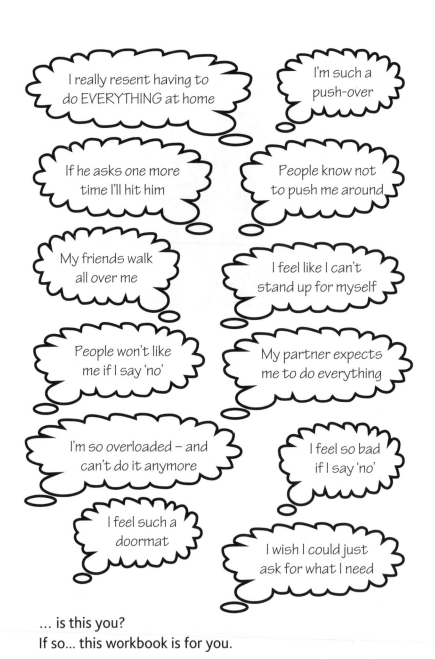

... is this you?

If so... this workbook is for you.

Overcoming Anxiety, Stress and Panic © Dr Chris Williams 2015

In this workbook you will:

- Learn about the differences between passive behaviour, aggressive behaviour and assertive behaviour.
- Learn the rules of assertion and how you can put them into practice in everyday situations.

What is assertiveness?

KEY POINT
Assertiveness is about being able to make sure your opinions and feelings are considered. You can be assertive without being forceful or rude.

Assertiveness means:

- Letting others know about your feelings, needs, rights and opinions while maintaining respect for other people.
- Expressing your feelings in a direct, honest and appropriate way.
- Realizing it's possible to stand up for your rights in such a way that you don't disregard another person's rights at the same time.

Assertion is **not about winning,** but about being able to walk away feeling that you put across what you wanted to say.

 Task

Try to think about a time when someone else has been assertive with you and respected your opinion.

 How did you feel about them and yourself?

About me – I felt:

About them – I felt:

Benefits of being assertive

Assertiveness is an **attitude** toward yourself and others that is helpful and honest. When you are being assertive, you ask for what you want:

- Directly and openly.
- Appropriately, respecting everyone's opinions and rights.
- Confidently, without undue anxiety.

By being assertive, you try not to:

- Disregard other people's rights.
- Expect other people to magically know what you want.
- Freeze with anxiety and avoid problems.

Being assertive improves your self-confidence and others' respect for you.

What do you do in difficult situations?

However confident you are, there are times when one finds it hard to deal with certain situations. For example:

- Dealing with unhelpful shop assistants.
- Planning to have *you* time away from your family.
- Asking for help when you need it.
- Asking someone to return something they have borrowed.
- Letting your family or friends know how you feel and what you need.
- Saying no to other people's demands.

Do you sometimes deal with these situations by losing your temper, by saying nothing or by **giving in**? If you do, have you noticed that it can leave you feeling unhappy, angry or out of control?

How can you become more assertive?

While growing up, people learn to relate to others from their parents, teachers and friends. You may also be influenced by other things such as TV and magazines. You may have read about how important it is to be a 'perfect' parent and do a great job of this all the time. But in trying to do this, you can become so focused on doing things for other people that you may forget to do things for yourself as well.

Sometimes a person's confidence can get worn away, for example if they have been bullied or ridiculed when they were growing up, or is criticized a lot by their family. In these situations, a person may learn **to react passively or aggressively** to people and situations.

> **KEY POINT**
> The good news is that although you may have learned to react passively or aggressively in life, you can become more assertive by learning **assertiveness skills**.

Key elements of passive behaviour

Behaving passively means:

- Always saying 'Yes'.

- Not letting others know about your feelings, needs, rights and opinions.

- Always choosing others' needs over your own.

Usually people behave passively to **avoid conflict** and to **please others**. This kind of behaviour is driven by a fear of not wanting to upset others, or having others not like us. But in the longer term, this can make you feel worse.

When you behave passively, others can take you for granted and increasingly expect you to drop everything to help them.

Key elements of aggressive behaviour

Aggression is the opposite of assertion.

Behaving aggressively means:

- Not respecting other people.

- Demanding things in an angry or threatening way.

- Thinking your own needs are more important than those of others. An aggressive person ignores other people's needs and thinks others have little or nothing to contribute.

The aim of aggression is to win, even at the expense of others.

Task

Overall, in the longer term, being aggressive causes problems for the person himself or for the people around him.

 KEY POINT
Behaving aggressively or being passive can be changed by learning the skill of 'assertive communication'.

So assertiveness means stating clearly what you expect and making sure that what you want is considered **as well as** what other people want.

You can **learn and practice** being assertive. By practicing being assertive, you'll become more aware of your own needs as an individual.

The rules of assertion

The following rules can help you live your life more assertively.

I can:

- Respect myself – who I am and what I do.
- Recognize my own needs as an individual, that is, separate from what's expected of me in particular roles, such as 'mother', 'brother', 'partner', 'daughter', 'son'.
- Make clear 'I' statements about how I feel and what I think, for example, 'I feel very uncomfortable with your decision'.
- Allow myself to make mistakes, recognizing that it's normal to make mistakes.
- Change my mind if I choose to.
- Ask for 'thinking about it time'. For example, when I'm asked to do something, I have the right to say 'I would like to think it over and I will let you know by the end of the week'.
- Allow myself to enjoy my successes, that is, being pleased with what I've done and sharing it with others.
- Ask for what I want, rather than hoping someone will notice what I want.
- Recognize that I am not responsible for the behaviour of other adults or for pleasing other adults all the time.
- Respect other people and their right to be assertive and expect the same in return.
- Say I don't understand.
- Deal with others without depending on them for approval.

Overcoming Anxiety, Stress and Panic © Dr Chris Williams 2015

At the moment, how much do you believe in each of these rules, and do you put them into practice?

I can:	Do you believe this rule is true?		Have you applied this in the last week?	
Respect myself	Yes ☐	No ☐	Yes ☐	No ☐
Recognize my own needs as an individual independent of others	Yes ☐	No ☐	Yes ☐	No ☐
Make clear 'I' statements about how I feel and what I think, for example, 'I feel very uncomfortable with your decision'	Yes ☐	No ☐	Yes ☐	No ☐
Allow myself to make mistakes	Yes ☐	No ☐	Yes ☐	No ☐
Change my mind	Yes ☐	No ☐	Yes ☐	No ☐
Ask for 'thinking about it time'	Yes ☐	No ☐	Yes ☐	No ☐
Allow myself to enjoy my successes	Yes ☐	No ☐	Yes ☐	No ☐
Ask for what I want, rather than hoping someone will notice what I want	Yes ☐	No ☐	Yes ☐	No ☐
Recognize that I am not responsible for the behaviour of others or for pleasing others all the time	Yes ☐	No ☐	Yes ☐	No ☐
Respect other people and their right to be assertive and expect the same in return	Yes ☐	No ☐	Yes ☐	No ☐
Say I don't understand	Yes ☐	No ☐	Yes ☐	No ☐
Deal with others without being dependent on them for approval	Yes ☐	No ☐	Yes ☐	No ☐

You can put these rights into practice to develop assertiveness skills by using many assertiveness techniques. Some of these are described below.

Before learning assertiveness techniques, it's sometimes also important to consider how to start a conversation.

Starting and maintaining conversations

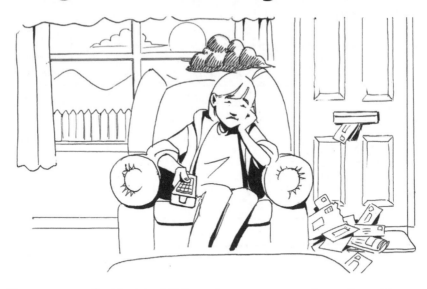

Sometimes you can feel isolated if there is no-one around to talk to. You may feel lonely but you lack contact with anyone. There are many practical things you can do to begin to meet people. For example:

- Making friends through people you know already.

- Joining an aerobics class or some other group sport at your local leisure centre, or a playgroup if you have small children.

- Taking a course, such as an adult evening class, to learn a new language, or joining a club, for example at your local community hall.

- Visiting other local places where you can meet others, for example community organizations or the local place of worship. Some local shops such as post offices, pharmacies and hairdressers also provide a place to talk.

- Getting in touch with people you knew but haven't seen for a while. Use e-mail, write a letter or telephone to get in touch. Arrange to meet if you can.

A key step in all of these ideas is that initial 'hello'. Things often flow easier once you have overcome that initial hurdle.

Here are some good conversation starters:

- How are you?

- Nice day isn't it?

- Hi, I'm new here and a little bit nervous.

- How old is your baby? He looks so alert.

Overcoming Anxiety, Stress and Panic © Dr Chris Williams 2015

You don't have to use these suggestions if you don't like them. Instead you can think of some other **conversation starters in advance**. Good opening questions often begin with the words:

- **What?** – What was the meeting like last week? What did you do yesterday? What was the new film like?

- **How?** – How did you find the meal? How are you? How are you getting on with the decorating?

- **When?** – When will we be covering this on the course? When do you start back at work?

- **Who?** – Who came yesterday? Who's that over there?

- **Why?** – Why does that happen (or not happen)? Why do we do things this way?

Follow these with **back-up questions** to keep the conversation going. For example:

- Who came yesterday – did they enjoy it?

- What did they say?

- Did it go well?

- Do you think they'll come back?

And of course, remember to listen!

Assertiveness techniques you could use

Once you get into conversation, the following techniques will help you to build assertive communication into what you say.

'Broken record'

First, practice what you want to say by repeating over and over again what you want or need. During the conversation, keep returning to your prepared lines, stating clearly what it is you need or want. Don't be put off by clever arguments or by what the other person says. Once you have prepared the lines you want to say, you can relax. This works in virtually any situation.

 Example: Being firm about what you want

Raj: 'Can I borrow £10 from you?'

Paul: 'I cannot lend you any money. I've run out.'

Raj: 'I'll pay you back as soon as I can. I need it desperately. You are my friend aren't you?'

Paul: 'I cannot lend you any money.'

Raj: 'I would do the same for you. You won't miss £10.'

Paul: 'I am your friend but I cannot lend you any money. I'm afraid I can't afford it just now.'

Remember

- Work out beforehand what you want to say.

- Repeat your reply over and over again and stick to what you have decided to say.

Saying 'no'

Many people find that 'no' seems to be one of the hardest words to say. Try to remember when you have found yourself in situations that you didn't want to be in, just because you avoided saying this one simple word.

Why does this happen? People often worry that they may be seen as mean and selfish, or they may worry about being rejected by others. This may prevent you from saying 'no' when you need to.

 KEY POINT
Saying 'no' can be both important and helpful.

 Task

Q Do I have problems saying 'No'?

Yes ☐ No ☐ Sometimes ☐

If you ticked 'Yes' or 'Sometimes', try to practice saying 'No' by using the following techniques:

- Be straightforward and honest so that you can make your point effectively. This isn't the same as being rude.

- Tell the person if you are finding it hard.

- Don't apologize and give all sorts of reasons for saying 'No'. It is okay to say 'No' if you don't want to do something.

- Remember that it is better in the long run to be truthful than breed resentment and bitterness within yourself.

Body language and assertiveness

How people communicate involves more than just words. Your voice tone, how quickly and loudly you speak, eye contact and body posture – all affect how you come over. When you're being assertive be aware of the nonverbal communications you make as well as the words you say.

Eye contact

- Meet the other person's eyes from time to time.

- Make eye contact – but don't stare at the person.

- Try not to look down for long – this may seem rude to others.

If you find this hard to do, practice looking just past the person. For example, look at a thing such as a picture on the wall behind the person. This shows you are paying attention – but without directly meeting the other person's eyes.

Your voice

- Try to vary your tone so you come over as interested and interesting.

- Don't be afraid of silence – especially if you've asked a question. When you ask a question you may be tempted to fill any uncomfortable gaps yourself. Be prepared to allow a little silence. Likewise, you don't need to reply instantly to any question. Remember that you're allowed some time to think.

- Think about how quickly or loudly you talk. Aim for a relaxed yet serious manner if you can.

Posture

Think about how you hold your body:

- Try looking up and don't hunch over – this can happen when you feel vulnerable or anxious.

- Keep an appropriate distance ('personal space') between you and the other person.

- Don't get too close – this might be seen as aggressive or inappropriate (unless you know the person very well).

Be friendly

Smiling and laughing once in a while is a friendly thing to do. People will often smile back. It has to be natural though and not forced (remember those politicians on TV).

Be relaxed in your body

- Think about how you hold your body. If you're tense or anxious you may clench your fists and frown, which may come over as being aggressive.

- Relax your body. Quickly think about how you are holding your arms and shoulders and try to relax tense muscles. Some people tend to pull up their shoulders toward their ears when they feel tense. Drop them down and relax.

A word of caution

Don't think you have to suddenly get all of this right straightaway. You should make these changes slowly – over many weeks or even months.

You shouldn't get too concerned about whether you are avoiding eye contact or smiling enough. All you need to do is be aware of this and try to occasionally make some small changes in what you do. Experiment and see what works for you.

Trying out being more assertive

Think about the following when you plan to respond assertively. Choose:

- **The right person**. Some people can take even assertive feedback badly. If you know that what you say is likely to be misinterpreted or that the person will overreact then you need to get some extra help, such as from a close friend or a family member.

- **The right time**. For example, try not to start talking about important things as soon as your partner gets in from work or from an evening out and is feeling tired or has been drinking. Choose a more relaxed time – or plan such a time – for example, go for a walk together.

- **The right issue**. The issue needs to be something that the other person can change. For example, asking your mother to look after your baby at times when she has to go to work is not realistic. Instead, choose a time that will suit you both.

- **The right words**. Use the approaches described in this workbook ('Broken record' and 'Saying no'). These techniques will help you to say what you need.

Summary

In this workbook you have learnt:

- The differences between passive behaviour, aggressive behaviour and assertive behaviour.
- About the rules of assertion and how you can put them into practice in everyday life.

Before you go

What have you learned from this workbook?

What do you want to try next?

Putting into practice what you have learned

Think about how you can be more assertive in your own life. If you recognize that you lack assertiveness, try to:

- Try out one of the two assertiveness techniques during the next week.

- Remind yourself about and put into practice the **rules of assertion**. Copy page the chart showing the rules of assertion earlier in this workbook or tear it out and carry it around with you. Put it somewhere you will see it (for example, by your TV or on a door or mirror or on the fridge) to remind you of these rules.

View this as an action plan that can help you to change how you are and also to learn something new about yourself and other people.

Plan, Do and Review

Whatever you choose to do, the first step is to make a plan and then try it out. The *Planner sheet* will help you create a clear and realistic plan. The next step is to use the *Review sheet* to consider how things have gone, and whether good or bad to learn from it. Copies of both sheets are found at the end of the workbook, and as with all the worksheets can be downloaded from www.llttf.com.

Other sources of support

 www.llttf.com (www.livinglifetothefull.com; Twitter @llttfnews)

This popular resource is designed to support readers of this course. There's also a forum where you can make comments, or ask questions of other people using the same course.

Acknowledgments

The cartoon illustrations were produced by Keith Chan, kchan75@hotmail.com.

The terms LLTTF and Five Areas are registered trademarks of Five Areas Resources Ltd.

Although we hope you find this book helpful, it's not intended to be a direct substitute for consultative advice with a healthcare professional, nor do we give any assurance about its effectiveness in a particular case. Accordingly, neither the publisher nor the author shall be held liable for any loss or damages arising from its use.

Planner sheet

1. *What* am I going to do?

2. *When* am I going to do it?

Write in the day and time:

3. Is my planned task one that:

Q Will be useful for helping me move forward?   Yes ☐   No ☐

Q Is clear, so that I will know when I have done it?   Yes ☐   No ☐

Q Is something that I value, or need to do?   Yes ☐   No ☐

Q Is realistic, practical and achievable?   Yes ☐   No ☐

4. What problems/difficulties could arise, and how can I overcome this?

What could get in the way? Write your possible blocks in here:

Do you need to rewrite your plan to tackle these possible blocks?

5. Write down your final plan here.

What are you going to do?

When are you going to do it? (day and time)

Your back-up plan: Think of another back-up solution you could turn to if for whatever reason there are problems with your plan.

KEY POINT
If you feel worse with symptoms you can still choose to do the planned activity anyway – because it's important.

Review sheet

What did you plan to do?

Write it here.

What happened? Did you attempt the task?   Yes ☐   No ☐

If yes:

● What went well?

● What didn't go so well?

● What have you learned about from what happened?

● How are you going to apply what you've learned?

If not:

What stopped you?

● *Internal factors* (e.g. forgot, not enough time, put it off, concerns I couldn't do it, I couldn't see the point of it, etc.)

● *External factors* (events that happened, work/home issues, etc.)

● How could you have planned to tackle these blocks?

Use the *Plan, Do, Review* approach to help you move forward.

Worksheets to help you practice *Being assertive*

Practice is important to help you master this approach. You can download worksheets of all of the key skills used in this workbook from:

www.llttf.com/worksheets/odlm

My notes

Building relationships with your family and friends

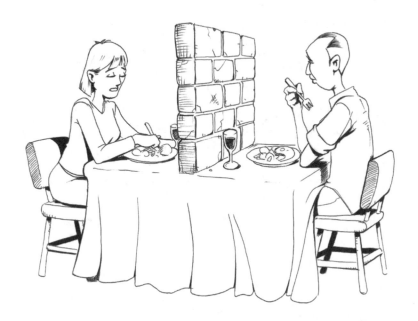

www.llttf.com or www.livinglifetothefull.com [t] @llttfnews (public)

www.fiveareas.com [t] @fiveareas (practitioners)

[f] www.llttf.com/facebook

Dr Chris Williams

overcoming
depression and low mood
a five areas approach

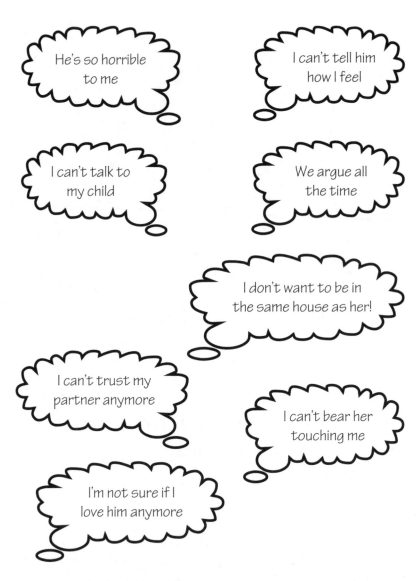

Are you feeling like this?

If you are... this workbook is for you.

In this workbook you will:

● Review your own style of communicating with others.
● Learn how to build (and rebuild) close relationships with the people around you.

The Five Areas and your relationships

You have learned about how low mood can affect you in each of the five areas of your life. Now use this same approach to think through how you feel can affect your relationships with those around you.

Relating to other adults

Some people have many friends and acquaintances. Others prefer to keep to themselves and are close to fewer people. Our past and present relationships have a powerful effect on how we feel. People tend to repeat the pattern or styles of relating that they learn in childhood. For example, during your upbringing, you learned important rules about:

● How you should communicate with others – with assertiveness, passivity or aggression.

● How you expect others to relate to you – whether they are trustworthy or will let you down.

How to deal with conflict and upset

Many of the rules people learn are helpful and positive. For example, that you are loved, trusted and accepted. However, sometimes the rules are negative and unhelpful.

> **KEY POINT**
> Most of us learn a mixture of both helpful and unhelpful rules and these can affect how you react to and trust others – especially when you are upset.

Use the checklist provided to find out your own styles of relating.

Repeating patterns in relationships

These rules explain why sometimes you repeat the same patterns in relationships. They help you understand why people always go for the same type of person and

What you may have learned from past experience	How this affects your relationships now (your relationship style)	Tick here if this applies to you – even if only sometimes
Learning generally positive things about how you see yourself, others and relationships	You mostly like yourself and have a good self-esteem. You generally think positively of others while realizing that you and they have faults. You are able to trust others, and make a commitment in relationships. This is a healthy state to be in and to aim for.	☐
Developing a low sense of worth/self-esteem. You doubt whether you can be loved. You may believe you are unattractive, boring or unlovable. You may fear that if others knew the real you they would run raway.	You put on a front and can't be yourself. You can be clingy and dependent in relationships and may passively do anything to keep a partner happy. You may use alcohol, drugs or sex because you think they make you more interesting.	☐
Developing a high, but fragile, self-esteem. You may have been taught as a child that you can do anything, that the whole world revolves around you. You see yourself as special. If there are problems, these are caused by others not you.	You can be very demanding of others. Everything must revolve around you. You need to get your own way. You are often impatient with others who don't see the point. You may seek out passive partners who will look up to you and do what you want. At the same time you may know you could always do better. Job titles and roles really matter. Yet you may quickly feel dissatisfied with jobs and people and want to move on.	☐
Thinking of yourself as ugly, unattractive or unlovable	You may feel uncomfortable and avoid close relationships and commitment to protect yourself from hurt ('It will never last'). You are uncomfortable being touched intimately by others. You may dress down and cover up any attractive features by wearing looser clothes. You may give up and let yourself 'go'. Or you may become obsessed that you must look 'just right'. You may flirt or sleep around to test whether you are really attractive, or you may constantly test the love of those who care about you – which frustrates and drives people away.	☐

Others are untrustworthy. You may have learned that people you love let you down or abandon you.	You may find it difficult to commit or respond with trust to others – even when they want to make a commitment to you. Your lack of trust may keep people at a distance.	☐
Sometimes your doubts can lead to jealous worries or anger.	Jealousy usually comes from fear and can severely damage your relationships. You may make demands that your partner never go out alone, especially with potential partners. You may accuse them of being attracted to others, or become obsessed and clingy so you suffocate and restrict them.	☐
Learning that others use you sexually. You may have learned that sex is something to just do, or have done to you. You may have been taught that sex is dirty or wrong, or it is about power/winning and getting your own way.	You may withdraw from the possibility of sex. You cannot enjoy this aspect of life or you use sex to get what you want. These rules may prevent you from developing a sex life where you can have trust, commitment and enjoyment. You may end up in patterns of relationship with partners who make demands and do not respect you.	☐
Learning not to show your emotions. You may have learned it's dangerous to show your emotions, or that being seen to be upset is a sign of weakness.	The stereotype is that men bottle up their emotions. They use drink or work to block how they feel. Women may be happier discussing their emotions and relationships with others. Of course both patterns can occur with either gender. What matters is the match (or mismatch) between two people. For example, when one partner feels distressed and is struggling to cope, they may desperately want to discuss issues but their partner may not want to. This clash of styles can lead to further difficulties.	☐

why they repeat mistakes. Being aware of these patterns is the first step towards changing them.

> **KEY POINT**
> Patterns and rules that might have made sense previously might not be so helpful now. You **can** learn new rules and new patterns of relationships.

Partners feeling they are being rejected

Being depressed changes your life. Partners often don't realize how they can feel squeezed out by the depression. Some partners understand what is happening and offer support and love. Others feel confused or hurt and withdraw or sulk or throw a tantrum. If you are feeling down, and especially if you are struggling, the last thing you need is a partner or spouse who is feeling touchy.

So if, for example, you don't feel like having sex (because of depression, or just because you may be tired), your partner may think that things are on the rocks and feel rejected. But first let's think some more about how **you** relate to important others around you.

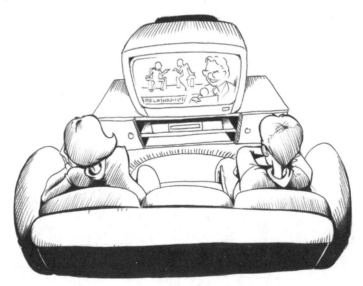

How do you relate to others you are close to?

The following questions will help you recognize your own attitudes and reactions towards the people you are close to. It may be tempting to answer these questions quickly with what you think of as the 'correct' answer, but take some time to think about your answers. The purpose of this task is to help you to recognize the things that may need to change for you to build more balanced relationships.

Q How do I respond to people I get close to – and how do they respond to me? Think back on your current and past close relationships including friendships.

Q What *helpful* relationship styles do you repeat? (Things you do that build closeness and respect.)

Q What *unhelpful* relationship styles do you repeat? (Things you do that damage closeness and reduce respect.)

Q How do these patterns affect your relationships – now and in the past?

Q How might these factors affect how you respond when you feel distressed?

Q Do you often feel uncomfortable when speaking about how you or someone close to you feels?

Q Do you try to avoid speaking about how you feel? How do those around you react to this?

> **KEY POINT**
> Unhelpful patterns may not affect you much of the time. However, they can come to the surface when you're feeling distressed. They then affect how you react to those around you.

What factors have shaped my attitudes and responses?

Think about the things from the past (your upbringing, childhood memories and comments that your parents, friends, others you respect, or people from popular culture have made) that affect how you approach intimate relationships.

 How has your own upbringing affected your view of how to relate to those you are close to?

Things you can do that can make a difference

The following are some things you can do (and not do) to build relationships.

With people you don't know so well (like neighbours or people you meet)

Do:

- Be yourself.

- Have planned a one-line statement if someone asks 'How are you?'. Remember, they don't know you well. They may not be aware you are finding things difficult at the moment. Don't feel you have to tell the person everything about yourself. Say something like 'Getting on fine thanks. How are you?', and leave it at that.

Don't:

- Tell everyone about every aspect of your life and how you feel – this is something you do with a therapist, other health worker or trusted friend.

With trusted friends and family members

Your wider family and friends can be a great support for you. A separate workbook, *Information for families and friends – how can you offer the best support?* – has been written for them. You might wish to show that workbook to them or go through it together.

Do:

- Seek out support from close friends.

Don't:

- Push people away and try to cope by yourself when you need help.

- Become overly focused on just one relationship, for example just one friend or just your baby.

- Confuse friendship and sex. Don't damage a good confiding friendship by something that 'just happened'.

With your partner/spouse or your girlfriend/boyfriend

Your partner/spouse or your boyfriend/girlfriend may be your closest support and companion, so this relationship can have a big effect on how you feel. Sometimes difficulties may arise and there may be anger, jealousy, boredom and affairs. These problems often are the result of a breakdown of communication and even love.

- **Communication**. Communication problems can happen in any relationship, but they are more difficult when you are low or stressed. You may not feel like talking for long, or giving or getting hugs or affection. Sometimes these changes are sudden, but more often they build up slowly over months or years. After a while you may find you have nothing to say. You may find it hard to even start a conversation. Your partner feels like a stranger.

- **Sex**. You may lose interest in sex or become anxious about whether you are still attractive.

- **The Internet**. You may develop a sense of emotional closeness with someone you are chatting with online. But be careful that this doesn't replace the closeness and support that people around you can offer. Some online options such as 'live flirting' or pornography will not only cost you money, but may also damage your real relationships by stopping you from committing emotionally. If you come across websites that you think would damage you emotionally, add them to your restricted zone on your Internet browser. Try actively to choose not to go back to them. Also, beware of the excitement and guilt that comes with Internet addiction.

- **Affairs**. Sometimes people try to jolt themselves out of a low mood by having a one-night stand or starting an affair. This may be caused by loneliness, low self-esteem or anger. Some people may use telephone sex lines, or dating agencies that promise 'discreet' relationships. Your partner may have reacted similarly.

- **Time apart**. A symptom of a relationship in trouble is often that we make choices to not be around each other. Do you make excuses to be elsewhere? Do you or your partner choose to work late, or go out without each other more? Sometimes people cope by throwing themselves into looking after their children. Children may provide some people the sense of emotional connection that is missing in their marriage/partner. People can drift apart even when they are in the same room, for example, never really talking while watching TV.

Ultimately these problems come down to the issues of **communication** and **commitment**. Even when feelings seem to have been lost for each other, often relationships can improve again given time, communication, forgiveness and commitment.

Rebuilding relationships with a partner/spouse by building communication and commitment

A key issue is how much change you both feel you need to make to improve things. To rebuild (or build) a relationship can sometimes come down to one partner making all the changes, but that misses the point of the need for *both* partners to discuss and work on their relationship problems together – if they both want to.

It may be that only some small changes of direction are needed. If so, some immediate things you can do together include:

- Listen – pay attention – don't just switch off and think you know what your partner is going to say. Talk about your day and ask about your partner's. Ask questions about the small but important details in life.

- Do things together – for example, spend time eating meals together as a family.

- Tackle 'relationship killers' such as always doing things apart.

- Anger and guilt can eat away at a relationship. You may need to forgive your partner – or ask for forgiveness from them if you have done things that have caused pain.

- Consider a regular 'date night' like you had early in the relationship.

- Develop physical intimacy in your everyday life at a level that you both feel happy with. Hugging, kissing and holding hands can build bridges. If you don't feel like having sex, try to discuss this. Try to agree that although you may not want to have sex as often (or even at all at the moment), you still might like hugs/kisses. Remember that even though you aren't interested in sex at the moment, your partner still has their sexual needs. Experiment and find activities that will satisfy both you and your partner's sexual needs.

- Bring back the romance – give surprises like a small gift, and compliments, or cook a nice meal. It's the thought and preparation time that matter here – not the cost. Extravagant gifts are no replacement for time together.

Hearing what we expect to hear

At the heart of many relationship problems is lack of communication. When people have drifted apart there is likely to be blame and hurt on both sides. When someone is distressed they can interpret things in extreme and unhelpful ways. This can strongly affect how two people interpret the same conversation.

People often think they know each other so well that **they think they already know what is going to be said**, so they don't listen to what is actually said. Sometimes they can be wrong.

 Example: Are you hearing what you expect to hear or are you listening to what is being said?

One partner may say something like 'That was a nice meal' and mean this as a compliment. However, because of suspicion and upset, their partner may hear it as 'Well you've cooked something nice for once – usually you don't make much effort.'

Sometimes people can be sarcastic when they offer compliments, but the danger is that positive or neutral replies may be interpreted in a negative way. Don't assume that others can read your mind. Sometimes you may not say what you really wanted to, and then feel upset when people don't act as you wan.t them to.

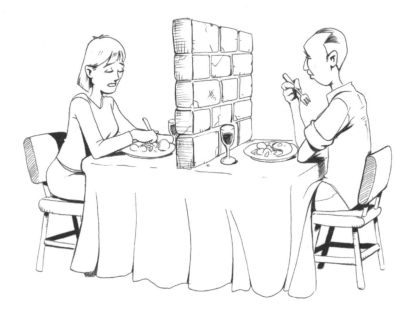

Task

Try this test to see if you both interpret the same event in the same way. Think about a time when you have both felt hurt, angry or upset. Then do this exercise when the heat has gone out. First complete the worksheet at the end of this workbook separately. Then compare what you have both written by answering the following questions:

Q How did the same situation affect how you both felt and what you did?

Q Do you both agree on exactly what happened?

Q Is there a difference in how you both see things?

Q Can this help explain your different reactions to this and other upsets?

Q Could this sort of different perception be happening again and again?

If miscommunication is an issue

First, decide that in future arguments you will both take stock and choose to clarify what the other is really saying rather than jumping to conclusions. Agree that if either of you isn't sure of what the other really means you will ask. But remember – ask politely and not in an angry or defensive way.

Try to rein in any immediate reactions if you feel upset, angry or hurt and instead **check it out**. If the other person is trying to be critical this will quickly come out, but often you may find that you've both got the wrong end of the stick. Sometimes when one or both of you are tired, or after having a drink, there may be more chance of miscommunication.

Some difficult issues

If your partner **feels like a total stranger** to you and you want to rebuild things, you both need to go back to the basics. Be open and discuss what you both want to do about things. If you both want to tackle this then agree on some ground rules about time together, sharing tasks and responsibilities, meal times, and sex. Slowly it is possible to rebuild feelings of love.

There may have been an affair, or awful things have been done or said, or **one of you may have moved out**. There may be a lot of hurting around. Again you both need to be open and discuss what you want to do about this. Can things recover – or is it too late?

Sometimes relationships end at this stage, in recrimination and anger – or just a sense of sadness. Sometimes they can move to friendship. Often things can still be rebuilt. Time can heal things. Counselling can help even very late in the day, but both people need to want to change things.

Violence and threats of violence

If you or a child is being abused, read this section

Men, women and children can be victims of abuse. It often leads to feelings of shame and isolation. If there is violence towards you or anyone else in the family then you need to be clear this is unacceptable. **If you or your child/children are being threatened or hit** you should think about leaving home – or ask your partner to leave at least for a time. Any violence or aggression is unacceptable. Children must be protected.

Many people feel powerless in violent relationships – or too scared to leave. If you are in this situation, you should seek professional help; for example, talk to your doctor or contact social services or the police. If you are scared to do this, tell a trusted friend and go with them. One thing you can be certain about is that unless things change, your relationship will be destroyed one way or another. Get the numbers of your **local domestic violence helplines** and support agencies. They are confidential and can give good advice.

If you are hitting/harming your partner or children

You need to recognize that hitting/harming your partner or children is unacceptable. This may be new behaviour as a result of anger linked to your depression or tension. Sometimes it's the effect of drinking. Violence and threats may be something that you have used for a long time. It's important that you recognize that you are hurting the people whom you love, and you must stop. Look for times when you are prone to losing control (for example when you are drinking) and work at responding differently.

You may find it helpful to join an anger management group. Your doctor can give you information about this. Reducing how much you drink can help and so can getting treatment for depression or anxiety. You will feel better for it – and you may be able to save and rebuild your relationship too.

Sometimes you need professional advice such as counselling to help rebuild your relationship.

KEY POINT
Ultimately, although many relationships can be rebuilt or lived with, sometimes they can't, and a time apart or permanent separation may result.

Summary
In this workbook you have:

- Reviewed your own style of communicating with others.
- Learned how to build (and rebuild close) relationships with the people around you.

Before you go

What have you learned from this workbook?

What do you want to try *next*?

Putting into practice what you have learned

Read or re-read the *Being assertive* workbook about the 'broken record' and 'saying no' approaches, and try to practice using them during the next week. In particular, the 'saying no' approach allows you to plan out how to be assertive in a particular situation and with a specific person. View this as an action plan that can help you to both change how you are and also learn something new about yourself and other people.

If relationships are a problem for you, consider showing this workbook to your partner. Read it through together. You might also want to go through the *Information for families and friends – how can you offer the best support* workbook.

Plan, Do and Review

Whatever you choose to do, the first step is to make a plan and then try it out. The *Planner sheet* will help you create a clear and realistic plan. The next step is to use the *Review sheet* to consider how things have gone, and whether good or bad to learn from it. Try to establish a routine of *Plan, Do* and *Review*. Copies of both sheets are found at the end of the workbook, and as with all the worksheets can be downloaded from www.llttf.com.

Other sources of support

 www.llttf.com (www.livinglifetothefull.com; @llttfnews)

This popular resource is designed to support readers of this course. There's also a forum where you can make comments, or ask questions of other people using the same course.

Acknowledgments

The cartoon illustrations were produced by Keith Chan, kchan75@hotmail.com.

The terms LLTTF and Five Areas are registered trademarks of Five Areas Resources Ltd.

Although we hope you find this book helpful, it's not intended to be a direct substitute for consultative advice with a healthcare professional, nor do we give any assurance about its effectiveness in a particular case. Accordingly, neither the publisher nor the author shall be held liable for any loss or damages arising from its use.

My thought review of a time when I felt worse

Please write in your thoughts in all Five Areas.

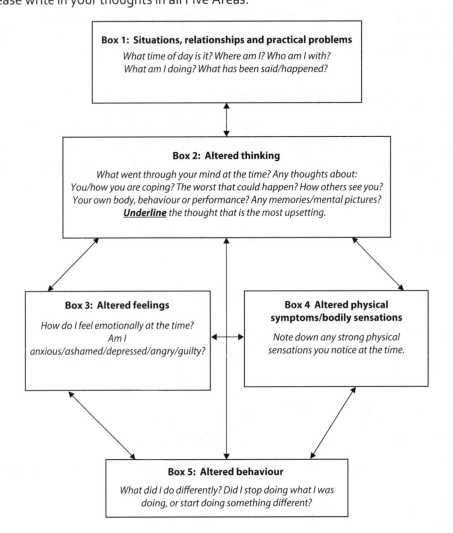

Box 1: Situations, relationships and practical problems

What time of day is it? Where am I? Who am I with?
What am I doing? What has been said/happened?

Box 2: Altered thinking

What went through your mind at the time? Any thoughts about:
You/how you are coping? The worst that could happen? How others see you?
Your own body, behaviour or performance? Any memories/mental pictures?
__Underline__ the thought that is the most upsetting.

Box 3: Altered feelings

How do I feel emotionally at the time?
Am I
anxious/ashamed/depressed/angry/guilty?

Box 4 Altered physical symptoms/bodily sensations

Note down any strong physical
sensations you notice at the time.

Box 5: Altered behaviour

What did I do differently? Did I stop doing what I was
doing, or start doing something different?

Planner sheet

1. *What* am I going to do?

2. *When* am I going to do it?

Write in the day and time:

3. Is my planned task one that:

Q Will be useful for helping me move forward?	Yes ☐	No ☐
Q Is clear, so that I will know when I have done it?	Yes ☐	No ☐
Q Is something that I value, or need to do?	Yes ☐	No ☐
Q Is realistic, practical and achievable?	Yes ☐	No ☐

4. What problems/difficulties could arise, and how can I overcome this?

What could get in the way? *Write your possible blocks in here:*

Do you need to rewrite your plan to tackle these possible blocks?

5. Write down your final plan here

What are you going to do?

When are you going to do it? (day and time)

Your back-up plan: Think of another back-up solution you could turn to if for whatever reason there are problems with your plan.

KEY POINT

If you feel worse with symptoms you can still choose to do the planned activity anyway – because it's important.

Review sheet

What did you plan to do?

Write it here.

What happened? Did you attempt the task?   Yes ☐   No ☐

If yes:

- What went well?

- What didn't go so well?

- What have you learned about from what happened?

- How are you going to apply what you've learned?

- **If not:**

What stopped you?

- *Internal factors* (e.g. forgot, not enough time, put it off, concerns I couldn't do it, I couldn't see the point of it, etc.)

- *External factors* (events that happened, work/home issues, etc.)

- How could you have planned to tackle these blocks?

Use the *Plan, Do, Review* approach to help you move forward.

Worksheets to help you practice *Building relationships with your family and friends*

Practice is important to help you master this approach. You can download worksheets of all of the key skills used in this workbook from:
www.llttf.com/worksheets/odlm

My notes

Information for families and friends – how can you offer the best support?

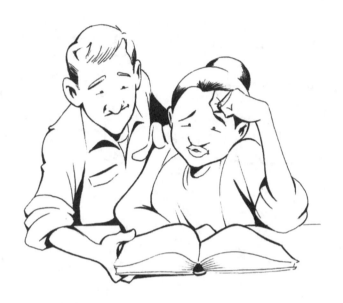

www.llttf.com or www.livinglifetothefull.com 🅴 @llttfnews (public)

www.fiveareas.com 🅴 @fiveareas (practitioners)

🅵 www.llttf.com/facebook

Dr Chris Williams

overcoming
depression and low mood
a five areas approach

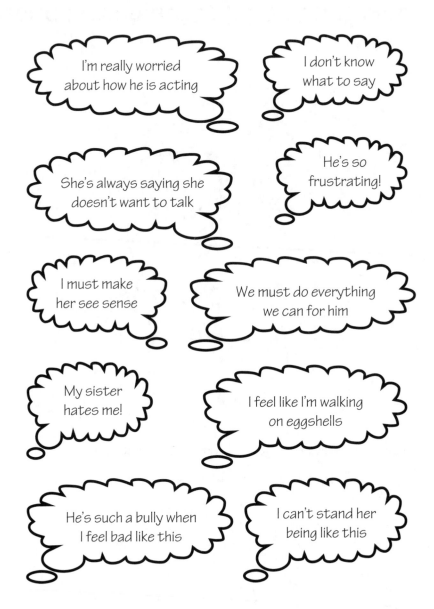

Are you feeling like this?

If so... this workbook is for you.

This workbook is for family and friends of people who are feeling unwell with low mood and depression. It also tells you more about the 'Overcoming depression and low mood' course so that family and friends can understand and offer support in the best possible way.

In this workbook you will learn about:

- What this course is about – and how the person you want to help is using it.
- Helpful things you can do so that you can offer the support that the person needs.
- Unhelpful things that you should avoid, which can undermine the support you can give.
- Looking after yourself as a friend or relative so that you stay well.
- Putting what you've learned into practice.

Background for friends and family

The course workbooks use a proven approach based on cognitive behavioural therapy (CBT, an action-oriented type of mental health therapy). CBT is known to work well for people who are facing many problems in their life – including stress and low mood. Research has confirmed that using the book with support is an effective treatment for depression.

An important part of your role is to provide support – and also an objective viewpoint. This can encourage the person and keep them on track while they try to work on their problems.

The approach used in the course looks in detail at five important areas of life. The **Five Areas™ assessment** helps a person recognize the kinds of problems they may be facing in each of the following areas:

1 Situations, relationships and practical problems involving the people and events around them

2 Their thinking (with extreme and unhelpful thinking)

3 Their feelings (emotions)

4 Their altered physical symptoms and bodily sensations

5 Their behaviour (any altered behaviour or activity levels)

> **KEY POINT**
> What we think about a situation or problem may affect how we feel emotionally and physically. It can also alter what we do.

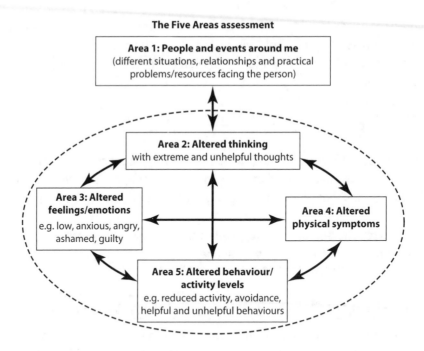

The Five Areas assessment

Because of the two-way links between each of the five areas, making helpful changes in any one of the areas can lead to benefits in the other areas as well. It also means that **the people around the person can help change things**.

About the workbook approach

The course workbooks aim to help people by:

- Providing useful information about how depression is affecting their life.

- Teaching important life skills to help make useful changes in the five areas of their life noted above.

The workbooks are practical, so the user has to apply the principles, not just read them. They are usually used one at a time – and the reader is encouraged to read them slowly. This allows them to practice what they have learned over a week or so before moving on to the next one. The person can discuss the workbooks (if they want) with others, such as family members, friends or a healthcare practitioner. Each workbook is the user's own resource and is private to them. Some people find it helpful to share them – but their wishes should be respected if they do not wish to share. The workbooks are like a personal diary, and as such they aren't meant to be read by everyone. However, this particular workbook is designed to be read and discussed jointly.

How can you help?

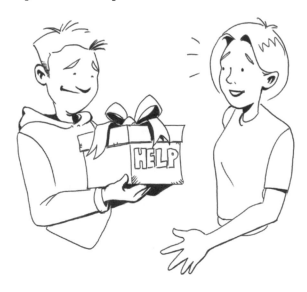

One of the most important things you can do is encourage the person you are help-ing to use the workbooks. This can be described as **supportive encouragement**. Support means:

- Being interested.

- Being hopeful as well as realistic.

- Encouraging the person to try things out – give it a go even if they feel bad at the time.

- Suggesting or freeing up a time when your friend or relative can use the materials. For example, if they have children, you can help by looking after them for an hour or so.

- Encouraging, not badgering. Ultimately each person must choose to do what they feel is important so that they can come to their own conclusion that it's useful to follow the plan even if they feel bad.

- Asking how you can help. Some people prefer to work alone or with someone other than a friend or family member, such as their health worker, who has a more neutral view.

It's important to remember that you are the friend or relative and not the therapist. Let the workbooks do the teaching and the therapeutic work. Your role is to help the person put what they are learning into action in their own life.

Other ways of supporting – keeping talking

When someone is struggling, family or friends may not fully understand what is going on or know how to offer help. Seeing each other's point of view at times like this is important. The danger is when either party starts to think that those around them no longer care. Stating clearly what you are thinking and feeling can really help move things forward.

You may have other worries. You may be concerned about the reactions of other people to your friend or relative's problem; for example, the attitude or comments of neighbours, colleagues, bosses, healthcare practitioners, people at your place of worship and other friends or relatives. When you've tried to help, you may have been uncertain how best to do this. You may struggle to know what to say. If you feel that you can't talk through things – or are unsure how either of you can show that you care – this workbook is for you.

Understanding the causes of low mood and depression

When a person breaks a leg, there is a large plaster cast on the leg to see. Physical conditions such as this are visible or can be picked up on scans of the body. But some symptoms aren't visible – for example, problems of tiredness, weakness, dizziness and pain. The same is true of feelings of sadness, stress and tension, which aren't visible in the same way as a broken leg, heart disease or cancer.

Some relatives and friends can't understand how a person can become depressed. They may think that there's no reason for the depression. But depression can strike anyone at any time for many reasons – physical, psychological and social. Even 'happy' events such as a holiday or having a baby can cause depression. The important thing is that whatever the cause of your friend or relative's depression, it is real to him or her, and you want to be there to help.

How to offer help

Complete the following checklist. It will help you recognize your friend or relative's strengths and it identifies possible problems that you may wish to tackle together. You might find it helpful to go through the checklist separately first, and then discuss your answers to each question together.

Can you identify any of these common problems that can arise for the sufferer?

- Isolation: your friend or relative finds it hard to talk to and receive support from others.

  Yes ☐   No ☐   Sometimes ☐

- There is no-one around who they can really talk to.

  Yes ☐   No ☐   Sometimes ☐

- You or others are unsure how to best offer support.

  Yes ☐   No ☐   Sometimes ☐

- You or others are avoiding talking about important symptoms and their impact.

  Yes ☐   No ☐   Sometimes ☐

- Perhaps even their healthcare practitioners may struggle to offer the kind of support needed.

  Yes ☐   No ☐   Sometimes ☐

- Are the symptoms not 'visible' or obvious to others?

  Yes ☐   No ☐   Sometimes ☐

- If 'Yes', does this seem to affect how others react?

  Yes ☐   No ☐   Sometimes ☐

Write down what you have both noticed here:

Avoiding things

When people feel anxious or worried, they may avoid certain situations, people, places, or even conversations that they feel may be difficult or stressful. This adds to their problems because although avoiding these things may allow a person to feel less anxious in the short term, in the long term avoidance can worsen the problem.

KEY POINT

The problem is that avoidance teaches you that the only way of dealing with a difficult situation is by avoiding it. Avoidance reduces your opportunities to find out that your worst fears don't occur. It worsens anxiety and strongly undermines confidence.

Example: Anne's and Mary's vicious circles of avoidance

Anne has arthritis and has been struggling to cope with her symptoms for several years. She finds it difficult to keep up with things in her flat or to get out and about.

Over the past few months Anne has felt increasingly low in mood. Her confidence has worsened and she can no longer cope with things. She tends to sit indoors, and cries from time to time. Her symptoms have been getting worse, and she feels she cannot enjoy many of the things that she used to.

Anne's sister Mary lives on the other side of town and likes to pop by once every week or so. A big problem for Anne is that she feels embarrassed when things aren't clean and neat in her flat, and when she isn't nicely dressed. So now whenever Mary calls by, Anne feels uneasy that Mary will notice that she isn't coping. She feels deeply ashamed of how things are and is very upset.

Mary is also concerned about Anne. She knows that Anne isn't being herself. They used to go out together from time to time and really enjoy doing things together. Now the 'spark' seems to have gone out of Anne.

Mary knows that Anne was badly affected when their brother and his family moved away earlier in the year. She wants to speak to Anne about how she wants to help. As a family they have always struggled with being open about how they feel. Although they love each other, this isn't something that is usually said, except perhaps in birthday and Christmas cards. Now whenever she visits Anne, Mary thinks, 'We should be discussing things – how can I help'. She has tried to bring up her concerns once or twice but Anne quickly becomes defensive and seems embarrassed.

Both Anne and Mary think, 'What can we do'?

Look at the two separate vicious circles of Anne's and Mary's avoidance.

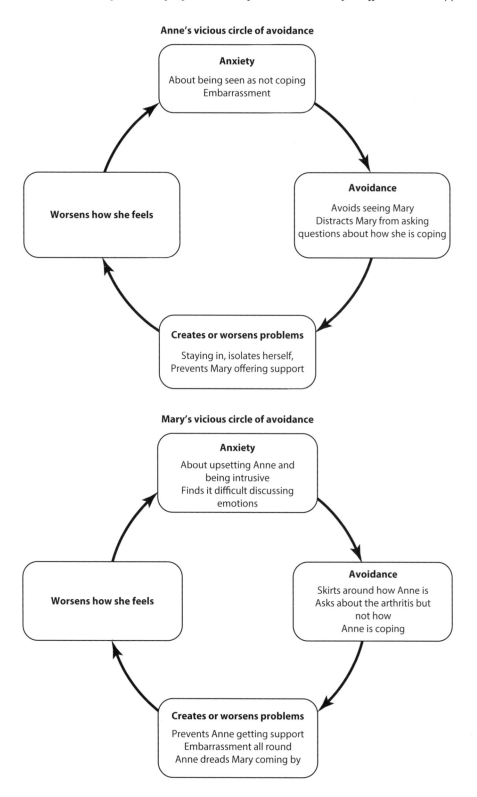

Anne's vicious circle of avoidance

Anxiety
About being seen as not coping
Embarrassment

Avoidance
Avoids seeing Mary
Distracts Mary from asking
questions about how she is coping

Worsens how she feels

Creates or worsens problems
Staying in, isolates herself,
Prevents Mary offering support

Mary's vicious circle of avoidance

Anxiety
About upsetting Anne and
being intrusive
Finds it difficult discussing
emotions

Avoidance
Skirts around how Anne is
Asks about the arthritis but
not how
Anne is coping

Worsens how she feels

Creates or worsens problems
Prevents Anne getting support
Embarrassment all round
Anne dreads Mary coming by

Task

Now answer the following questions:

Q How are Anne and Mary's reactions worsening the situation?

Q What could they do to change things?

As the example shows, sometimes even just *talking about the symptoms* can become something to be avoided at home or with friends. Even among close relatives and friends, a person may feel embarrassed about discussing such things.

 Task

The checklist below describes common areas of avoidance.

Family and friends checklist: identifying the vicious circle of avoidance

As a friend/family member, are you:	Tick here if you have noticed this – even if just sometimes
Avoiding asking about anything to do with low mood or depression?	☐
Avoiding talking to anyone else about your friend or relative's symptoms or about how they are coping?	☐
Putting off all decisions until the person is better? For example, putting holidays or other life plans completely on hold?	☐
Not really being honest? For example, saying 'Yes' when you really mean 'No'?	☐
Trying hard to avoid situations that bring about upsetting thoughts/ memories?	☐
Brooding over things and therefore no longer living your own life to the full?	☐
Avoiding discussing how you yourself are feeling or coping?	☐

(Continued)

Avoiding people/isolating yourself from others?	☐
Avoiding expressing concerns about how children in the family are doing if there is a clear problem here? If there is, it's important to make sure the care that is needed is given.	☐
Avoiding being assertive about your own needs?	☐
Avoiding going out in public either by yourself or with the person you are supporting?	☐
Avoiding being at home-keeping so busy that you don't have to think about the problem?	☐
For partners/spouses: If you are the person's partner/spouse, are you avoiding sex or physical intimacy? Perhaps you have fears of causing over-exertion or harm? Or perhaps you're not sure whether this would be imposing/inappropriate or not wanted at present?	☐

 Are you avoiding things in other ways?

If this is so, write down here how you are doing:

Sometimes, some of these questions can be hard to discuss. This may especially be true around issues such as sex or intimacy. You can always decide to discuss them at a later time but don't ignore them as they are important.

Remember that at times the avoidance can be quite subtle; for example, choosing to steer conversations away from difficult areas that would actually benefit from being discussed. Often people fear upsetting the other person or making them feel worse. This can backfire, however, because it means issues aren't dealt with.

Overcoming avoidance with clear communication

The only way of overcoming avoidance is with openness and honesty. If you are someone who worries about hurting other people's feelings, or aren't quite sure how to discuss things openly, then you might find the *Being assertive* and *Building relationships with your family and friends* workbooks helpful.

Building relationships

Here are some practical phrases and strategies you can use to relate to each other in a more positive way.

- Sometimes it can be helpful to say, 'This isn't a good time to talk, let's talk about it later.'

- Sometimes a person may need to work through an issue by talking at length. Let them talk – often no comment is needed. Listen for the main message, and then pick up on this point so they know you are really listening; for example, 'It sounds like you feel frustrated/fed up today...'.

- Offer praise and encouragement to build confidence; for example, 'I can see such a difference from a month ago...'.

- Look for things you can comment positively about (e.g. 'That dress looks really nice on you' or 'The children really enjoyed playing that game with you').

- Try to find at least three positive things to say every day.

Helpful and unhelpful responses

When someone you care about needs your help you try to improve things. Mostly, your responses are *helpful*. Sometimes however – without meaning to – how you react can be *unhelpful*. This section focuses on both the helpful and possible unhelpful behaviours of friends/relatives/carers.

Helpful activities by family and friends

- Finding out about depression; for example, by reading the workbooks in this course or other information booklets, getting information from self-help groups or getting information from healthcare practitioners. This can equip you with the knowledge and skills you need. Looking at the online course at **www .livinglifetothefull.com** (or **www.llttf.com**) may be helpful. (This is an added resource to support users of this workbook.)

- 'Being there' for the person for the long term.

- Being willing to talk and offer support when needed.

- Encouraging the person to ask questions of experts such as their GP or health visitor.

- Encouraging the person to put what they are learning into practice.

- Realizing there are no quick fixes.

- Using your sense of humour to help you and the person you support to cope.

Overcoming Anxiety, Stress and Panic © Dr Chris Williams 2015

- Planning time for yourself as well as for others.

- Using effective coping strategies to deal with your own feelings of tension.

- Looking after yourself.

- Seeing a healthcare practitioner for advice if you are struggling to cope.

- Pacing recovery. Recovering from depression takes time. Even when mood improves, there is a period (weeks to months) when a person is vulnerable to relapse. Think about the broken leg again. When the plaster comes off, you wouldn't expect a person to run a marathon the next day. Muscles need to be built up again. In the same way, although the depression may lift, a person needs to build up their confidence and activities slowly again. Helping them pace their recovery is one of the best ways of reducing the risk of relapse.

 Are you doing anything else that is helpful?

Unhelpful behaviours by family and friends

Sometimes family and friends think that they are doing something helpful when it's actually part of the problem. For example, wrapping the person in cotton wool, taking over everything from them, or bullying and forcing them to do something. Sometimes carers can also react out of frustration to 'let off steam'. Although this can make you feel better initially, it can backfire and create further problems. For example, some people may find that raising their voice in frustration can make them feel a lot better to begin with. But this can have a damaging effect on your relationship and leave you feeling guilty.

 KEY POINT
The hallmark of a truly helpful activity is that it's good for both you and for others.

No matter how helpful something may seem to begin with, if taken to an extreme most responses can backfire and become a problem. For example, seeking support from others is sensible. A problem shared can really help – but if you find that your friend or relative is constantly on the phone and feels they can't cope without talking to others then something that was originally helpful has become a problem.

Other unhelpful behaviours may include:

- Offering 'helpful advice' all the time.

- Trying to do everything for the person.

- Constantly offering reassurance that everything will work out fine ('Of course you'll be okay').

- Overly protecting and suffocating the person by taking away all their responsibility (and all their choices too).

People behave in this way for many reasons. Often it's due to concern, friendship and love. It may be the result of anxiety or guilt. Whatever the cause, when people offer too much help and want to do everything for another person, their actions can backfire and make things worse.

Frustration and anger at healthcare practitioners

It isn't unusual that when someone takes on a supportive or carer role they can struggle themselves. Feelings such as demoralization, worry, guilt, frustration and anger can occur. These frustrations can spill over into critical comments about healthcare practitioners looking after the person you care for.

It can be tempting to be critical, but most healthcare practitioners can offer helpful support. However, sometimes even those working in the caring professions may not be able to offer the kind of support that you feel your friend or relative needs.

KEY POINT
If you are too critical of healthcare practitioners, there is a danger that you will undermine the support and advice that they can offer.

But what if you disagree?

Sometimes people have strong opinions about what treatments or investigations their friend or relative whom they are supporting may need. For example, a person may have strong opinions about alternative and complementary medicine approaches, or they just may not feel the current treatment is working. They may have understandable worries about medication, for instance during pregnancy or while breastfeeding.

Overcoming Anxiety, Stress and Panic © Dr Chris Williams 2015

If your friend or relative is offered treatments or investigations that you have concerns about, it's important to be aware of how you respond. If they have been prescribed medication do not try to persuade them to suddenly stop taking their medication without discussing it with their doctor. If you have strong concerns that a treatment is wrong or is not needed, it's best for you to go along with the person (if they are agreeable to this) to the doctor to discuss it. What all of you want is the best possible outcome. It is important to remember that clinical depression is a serious problem and needs treatment in the same way as other serious illnesses.

 Task

Look at the following list of common unhelpful behaviours. Tick any activity you have found yourself doing over the last month.

Family and friends checklist: unhelpful behaviours

As a friend/family member, are you:	Tick here if you have noticed this – even if just sometimes
Becoming overly protective of the person – wrapping them in cotton wool?	☐
Taking over all responsibility from the person? For example, making all the important decisions, or trying to control every aspect of their life.	☐
Taking over all activities they used to do, so they don't have to 'worry' about them?	☐
Not allowing the person to be upset or distressed?	☐
Having a go at the person from time to time – through frustration or anger?	☐
Becoming so focused on the distressed person that other people's needs aren't met? For example, your own or other family members such as children are overlooked.	☐
Depending on or needing the sufferer to be well and functioning? (So that they aren't allowed to be unwell)	☐
Making snap decisions about important issues? For example, resigning a post to look after the person.	☐
Automatically advising the person not to try recommended treatment approaches because of your fears that it may do harm?	☐

Undermining or criticizing healthcare practitioners? (Because they haven't been able to find a cure)	☐
Helping the person avoid doing things because of fears about what harm might result? For example, taking over going to shops, or taking on all the driving. (This then further undermines their confidence)	☐
Constantly reassuring the person to allay their anxious fears?	☐
Constantly asking about how they are? (Which unhelpfully draws attention to illness)	☐
Speaking for/over the person in social settings, or in hospital outpatients, etc.? For example, you tell their story rather than them.	☐

 Write down any other unhelpful behaviours here:

 Overall: what effect do any unhelpful behaviours have on you both?

The problem is that these responses can quickly become a habit, and the same pattern is repeated again and again.

Wrapping the person in cotton wool

Offering extra special attention and support can also become unhelpful. The relationship may feel suffocating and frustrating. The person can end up feeling treated like a child. Although in such situations you may mean well, your actions can undermine your relationship.

When your friend or relative is trying to cope with symptoms, it's important to encourage them to keep as active as possible within the confines of what is reasonable for them. They should be encouraged to do everyday activities even though the symptoms are there – within the confines of what they physically are able to manage. If you take responsibility for doing everything, the danger is that they won't be as active as they could otherwise be and so you create unnecessary dependency.

Faith and seeking help

Carers may have a strong spiritual belief. This may be helpful, but these beliefs may emphasize prayer as the **only** way toward recovery and healing, which may undermine other methods of getting help.

People can tend to ignore the fact that health workers may have an important part in the recovery process, and their input may be part of an answer to prayer. In the same way that you would recommend someone seek medical help if they broke their arm or leg, a person should seek medical help for low mood and depression. If you have doubts about how the medical profession can help low mood and depression, please discuss your concerns with a spiritual leader whom you respect.

Staying well yourself

When you support others, you also need to look after yourself and allow time and space for your own needs. Depression and stress are very common among carers. You may be so busy offering support that you have no time for yourself.

Some methods of looking after yourself include:

● Having an open discussion about your own stress – for example, with trusted friends or relatives or within a carer support group.

● Taking short breaks/holidays/weekends away with others.

● Planning 'me time' such as hobbies/interests into the day and week.

● Seeing your own doctor to discuss the need for additional treatment and support.

When to get extra help

Although the person with depression has someone like you to support them during their illness, there are times when this won't be enough. You should support your friend or relative to get extra help if you think they have any of the following:

● **Severe depression**; for example continuing low mood, tearfulness, a serious lack of sleep or concentration, or a marked loss of weight or energy despite attempts to improve things.

● Strong urges to **self-harm,** feeling **hopeless** or having **suicidal** thoughts.

● Other **dangerous behaviours**; for example risk-taking, threats of harm to others.

- A possibility of immediate or longer-term significant harm or injury by an abusive partner or carer. For example, **abuse or neglect, including concerns for the health or safety of any children**.

- **Severe withdrawal from life activities**; for example they are clearly not coping well at all.

- **Severe weight loss** or the person has stopped drinking fluids and becomes dehydrated.

In these and other situations where extra help is needed or can be a real help and, if in doubt, it's important to ask for help in *deciding* whether more help is needed.

If there is a risk of immediate significant harm (abuse of others, self-harm or suicide), immediate action needs to be taken. At such times, professional and voluntary services can give a great deal of support.

What if the person doesn't agree they need extra help?

It is always best to get the person's agreement for getting extra help, but sometimes the risks involved may preclude this. If you are seriously worried that extra help is needed but the person is refusing, it's still best to ask for help in deciding if anything else can or should be done. Contact local health or social services. You can discuss the issues in confidence and will receive sensible advice.

KEY POINT

If you are worried or concerned, it is better to ask for help or advice than do nothing.

Summary

In this workbook you have learned:

- What this course is about – and how your friend or relative is using it.
- How best to help and communicate effectively.
- Helpful things you can do so that you can offer effective support, and unhelpful things to avoid.
- How to look after yourself and stay well.

Before you go

 What have you learned from this workbook?

 What do you want to try *next*?

Putting into practice what you have learned

You are likely to make the most progress if you can put into practice what you have learned in the workbook.

Continue to put into practice what you learn over the next few weeks. Don't try to tackle everything all at once. Plan out what to do at a pace that's right for you. Build changes one step at a time.

Building helpful behaviours and reducing unhelpful behaviours

To successfully plan a reduction in unhelpful behaviours or to increase helpful behaviours, you need to have a clear plan.

Do:

- Think how to slowly alter what you do step by step.
- Plan to alter only one response you make over the next week.
- Make changes one step at a time until you reach your eventual goal.
- Write down your plan in detail so that you will be able to put it into practice this week.

Don't:

- Choose a goal that is too ambitious to start with.

- Try to alter too many things at once.

- Be negative or think 'Nothing can be done, what's the point, it's a waste of time.' Try to experiment to find out if your negative thinking is accurate or helpful.

You will find a structure for how to plan ways of building helpful behaviours, over-coming reduced activity or avoidance, and reducing unhelpful behaviours in other workbooks in this course.

Try to learn from any mistakes and keep practicing, so that using this approach becomes second nature whenever you face a problem or you want to help your friend or relative.

Plan, Do and Review

Whatever you choose to do, the first step is to make a plan and then try it out. The *Planner sheet* will help you create a clear and realistic plan. The next step is to use the *Review sheet* to consider how things have gone, and whether good or bad to learn from it. Copies of both sheets are found at the end of the workbook, and as with all the worksheets can be downloaded from www.llttf.com.

Other sources of support

 www.llttf.com (www.livinglifetothefull.com; @llttfnews)

This popular resource is designed to support readers of this course. There's also a forum where you can make comments, or ask questions of other people using the same course.

Acknowledgments

The cartoon illustrations were produced by Keith Chan, kchan75@hotmail.com.

The terms LLTTF and Five Areas are registered trademarks of Five Areas Resources Ltd.

Although we hope you find this book helpful, it's not intended to be a direct substitute for consultative advice with a healthcare professional, nor do we give any assurance about its effectiveness in a particular case. Accordingly, neither the publisher nor the author shall be held liable for any loss or damages arising from its use.

Planner sheet

1. *What* am I going to do?

2. *When* am I going to do it?

Write in the day and time:

3. Is my planned task one that:

Will be useful for helping me move forward?	Yes ☐	No ☐
Is clear, so that I will know when I have done it?	Yes ☐	No ☐
Is something that I value, or need to do?	Yes ☐	No ☐
Is realistic, practical and achievable?	Yes ☐	No ☐

4. What problems/difficulties could arise, and how can I overcome this?

What could get in the way? Write your possible blocks in here:

Do you need to rewrite your plan to tackle these possible blocks?

5. Write down your final plan here

What are you going to do?

When are you going to do it? (day and time)

Your back-up plan: Think of another back-up solution you could turn to if for whatever reason there are problems with your plan.

KEY POINT
If you feel worse with symptoms you can still choose to do the planned activity anyway – because it's important.

Review sheet

What did you plan to do?

Write it here.

What happened? Did you attempt the task?   Yes ☐   No ☐

If yes:

● What went well?

● What didn't go so well?

● What have you learned about from what happened?

● How are you going to apply what you've learned?

If not:
What stopped you?

● *Internal factors* (e.g. forgot, not enough time, put it off, concerns I couldn't do it, I couldn't see the point of it, etc.)

● *External factors* (events that happened, work/home issues, etc.)

● How could you have planned to tackle these blocks?

Use the *Plan, Do, Review* approach to help you move forward.

Worksheets to help you practice *Information for families and friends – how can you offer the best support?*

Practice is important to help you master this approach. You can download worksheets of all of the key skills used in this workbook from:
www.llttf.com/worksheets/odlm

My notes

Doing things that boost how you feel

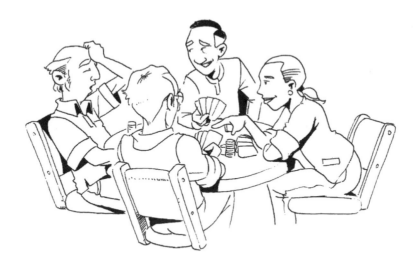

www.llttf.com or www.livinglifetothefull.com @llttfnews (public)

www.fiveareas.com @fiveareas (practitioners)

www.llttf.com/facebook

Dr Chris Williams

overcoming
depression and low mood
a five areas approach

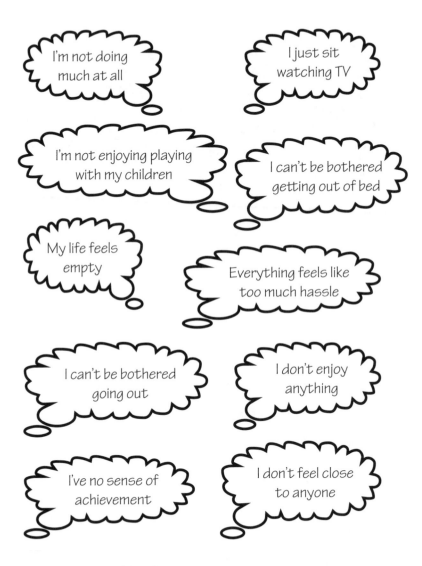

Are you feeling like this?

If so... this workbook is for you.

In this workbook you will:

- Learn how low mood and stress cause you to do less.
- Find out how reduced activity affects you.
- Discover what activities give you a boost.
- Identify things you have cut down or stopped doing which you used to enjoy.
- Start to rebuild a pattern to your day – and plan to tackle key essential tasks.
- Plan ways to make slow, steady changes to your life to boost how you feel – even if sometimes it feels hard.
- Choose to live life in a way that fits with your values.
- Plan some next steps to build on these changes.

How low mood can affect you

Depression makes life seem difficult because of:

- Low energy and tiredness ('I'm just too tired').

- Low mood – so you don't really enjoy things.

- Little sense of achievement – you feel as if you are on a never-ending treadmill.

- Loss of a sense of closeness to others. Instead of feeling happiness and love with your family and friends, you may just feel numb.

- Symptoms such as pain or weakness that can grind you down and make it harder to keep going.

- Negative thoughts about doing things ('I just can't do it').

So **you do less and less**. And when you do less, it can make you feel even worse. The less you do the worse you feel, and the worse you feel the less you do.

Many people try to force themselves to do things they feel *have* to be done – looking after children, working, doing chores. However, activities you would usually do for fun or friendship slowly get squeezed out. Even when you are active you may become so focused on just surviving that you don't have time to sit back and feel a sense of achievement in what you do.

How inactivity can affect you physically

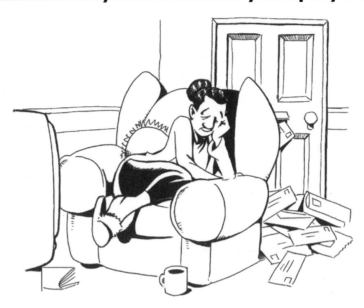

Being less active makes you feel physically worse. If you sit for a long time you can feel stiff, and your unused muscles weaken – adding to the vicious cycle of reduced activity.

The good news is that a slow, steady increase in activity can help improve your physical flexibility and reduce pain you may have from being sedentary. This is why physiotherapists and doctors advise people to increase activity levels. It can also boost your mood.

Example: Anne's reduced activities

Anne has arthritis. For years she has walked to the park and sat on the bench, and enjoyed chatting to people cycling and walking past. She loves listening to the radio and reading. She has a few good friends, and keeps in close contact with her brother Jake and her sister Mary. She is especially fond of Jake's children.

However, Jake and his family have moved away. Although they talk to Anne on the phone, it isn't the same. For the last six months Anne has struggled with worsening arthritis pain and is increasingly low and upset. She has stopped reading, listening to the radio and going to the park. She sits alone in her chair all day, and her back and legs have started to feel stiff, making it difficult for her to get out walking.

Overcoming Anxiety, Stress and Panic © Dr Chris Williams 2015

Now think about your own life.

 Have you reduced your activities? Write what you haven't been doing below.

- Overall, have you stopped doing things you used to enjoy because of how you feel?

Yes ☐   No ☐   Sometimes ☐

Has the reduced activity:

- Removed things from your life that previously gave you pleasure?

Yes ☐   No ☐   Sometimes ☐

- Has it worsened how you feel physically?

Yes ☐   No ☐   Sometimes ☐

Overall, has this worsened how you feel?

Yes ☐   No ☐   Sometimes ☐

If you have answered 'Yes' or 'Sometimes' to all the questions above, then reduced activity is causing a problem for you. This workbook will help you learn to overcome reduced activity.

Rebuilding your routine

One of the first things affected during low mood is your regular routine. Because things feel harder to do, you focus on just getting by. So you start to lose the structure to your day. All those routine things you took for granted can start to be lost:

- Getting up at a regular time.
- Washing your hair and bathing/showering each day.
- Eating regular meals and cooking food.
- Getting out working/meeting people.
- Going to bed at a regular time.

It is important to rebuild the pattern to your day to help you feel better.

First steps to boosting how you feel

The plan is to discover:

- The things you've done in the past that made you feel good.

- The things you are doing now that give you a boost.

- Ways of rebuilding your routine/pattern to the day.

- Key essentials that, if you don't do them, will cause you problems (for example not paying bills).

So you need to keep a **record** of the activities you are currently doing.

What activities should you record?

Use the *My Activity* sheets at the end of the workbook to record **everything** that you do over the next few days. For example:

- Getting dressed, washed/showered

- Doing housework or going out shopping

- Listening to the radio

- Going to work

- Having breakfast

- Chatting with your partner

- Doing the washing up

Also include times when you are sitting and watching TV, or resting, etc. Try to record **everything** – you are probably doing far more than you thought. For an example of a completed diary, see Anne's activity sheets later in this chapter.

Rating your activities

Using the graph below, rate your activities:

1. The **pleasure** or **fun** you have while doing the activity (0–10 scale).

2. How much you value the activity (0–10 scale).

3. How **close** you felt to people during the activity.

Doing this will help you understand what's good in your life, and what's missing.

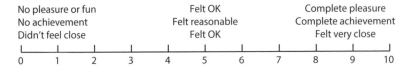

No pleasure or fun	Felt OK	Complete pleasure
No achievement	Felt reasonable	Complete achievement
Didn't feel close	Felt OK	Felt very close

0   1   2   3   4   5   6   7   8   9   10

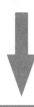

Example: Anne rates her activities

Anne goes out for a walk with her sister Mary, and gives this a score of 5/10 for pleasure. She also rates this activity as 7/10 for value to her (she didn't want to go, but managed it because she sees it as important to stay in touch to her sister). She also rates herself as 8/10 for closeness as she felt closer to Mary again as they chatted.

Anne's diary shows that even though she is doing less than she used to, she is still doing some things. Importantly, several of these activities can help her feel better. The key is to build on this to improve how she feels.

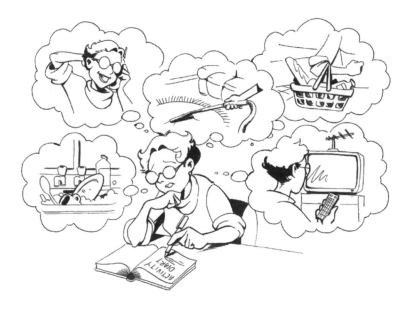

Example: Anne's activity sheets (morning and part-afternoon)

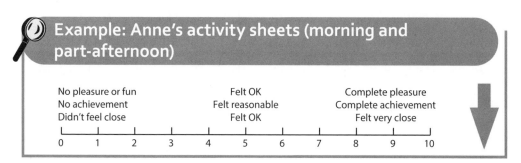

No pleasure or fun
No achievement
Didn't feel close

Felt OK
Felt reasonable
Felt OK

Complete pleasure
Complete achievement
Felt very close

0 1 2 3 4 5 6 7 8 9 10

Anne's activity

Date and time	Activity (include everything you do)	How long did you do it for?	Pleasure felt 0 = no pleasure 10 = maximum pleasure	What is the value/importance to you of the activity 0 = not important at all 10 = maximum importance	Sense of closeness to others 0 = no sense of closeness 10 = maximum sense of closeness
Morning	In bed, asleep	7 hours before this	/	/	/
8–9	Woke up and listened to music on the radio	30 minutes	5	2	3 – he's my favourite DJ
	Got up and had a shower, cleaned my teeth	40 minutes	3	6	1
	Made a coffee and had some toast	15 minutes	5	5	5
	Sat and rested for a time	60 minutes	0	0	7
Afternoon	Watched TV	50 minutes	5	2	2
	Did the ironing	45 minutes	6	8	2
	Mary called by, made her a drink	60 minutes	6	8	8

Task

Now start completing your activity sheets for the next few days. Use the blank Activity sheets diary at the back of this workbook, or copy it. You can download more for free from **www.llttf.com**. Don't forget to include what you're doing at the moment – reading the workbook.

Use your diary to discover **patterns** in what you do and don't do. Think about what it says about a routine pattern to your day. Also, are there any big things you should be doing that you are putting off?

Later, you will also use the diary to help you work out a first target to change.

 KEY POINT
Keeping a diary can help you find out which activities or situations make you feel better.

How the activity diary can help you move forward

The all-or-nothing approach

Overdoing things can sometimes be just as unhelpful as under-doing. This is called the **all-or-nothing** response. People may throw themselves into things on days when they feel better. The problem is that they may then crash back and feel worse. So on average they do less and less – as shown by the dotted line in the graph below.

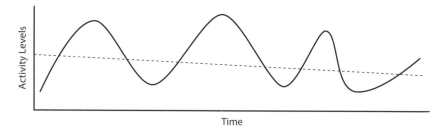

Time

 For example, if you are ironing the clothes:

- Taking a paced approach would include a break halfway through and maybe finishing later that day.
- Taking an 'all-or-nothing' approach would mean that you throw yourself into doing it all at once – exhausting yourself in the process.

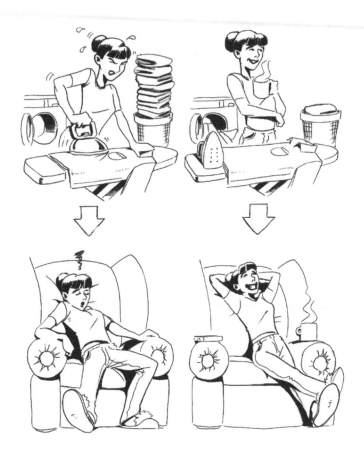

Choosing activities to do

Once you have an idea of your current activity level, you can build on this to pace yourself and increase your activity levels. Choose to do things that improve how you are mentally and physically by choosing activities that:

- Give you a sense of pleasure

- You value and see as important so you feel a sense of achievement

- Help you feel close to others

You will use the same activity sheets to plan what you will do. This can also help you **re-set a routine** to your day. Try to build in basic activities such as getting up, washing, eating healthy meals, meeting others/working and going to bed. Plan to build activities into your life across each day (morning, afternoon and evening).

Setting targets can help you make the changes needed to feel better. To do this you will need to decide:

- **Short-term** targets – Changes you can make today, tomorrow and the next week.
- **Medium-term** targets – The changes to be put in place over the next few weeks.
- **Long-term** targets – Where you want to be in six months or a year.

Identifying some targets for change

By now, you will have an organized idea of the activities you are doing – and not doing – from your activity sheets. This will help you identify some things you would like to do more of. Your sheets might not include all the things you like to do, so look through the list below and tick the ones that apply to you – the things you used to enjoy, but have cut down or stopped doing because of how you feel.

You will probably have noticed changes in at least some of these.

Checklist: identifying your patterns of reduced activity

As a result of how you feel, are you:	*Tick here if you have noticed this – even if just sometimes*
Getting up and going to bed at a regular time?	☐
Stopping or reducing doing hobbies or other things you previously enjoyed or did to relax?	☐
Going out or meeting friends less than usual?	☐
Eating poorly (for example eating less or eating more 'junk' food)?	☐
Noticing physical consequences of reduced activity – such as worsened pain or restricted joint movement?	☐
Brooding over things or just sitting watching TV?	☐
Not working or doing things that you value and see as important, such as helping others?	☐
Failing to keep up with housework ?	☐
Not always answering the phone or the door when people visit?	☐
Putting off things you should do, such as leaving letters/bills unopened or not replying to them?	☐

Continued

Paying less attention to your self-care (for example washing less, less bothered about your appearance, not shaving)?	☐
Enjoying or playing a sport?	☐
Gardening?	☐
Playing a musical instrument/singing?	☐
Reading a good book or watching a film?	☐
Less interested in sex (for example pushing your partner away because of a lack of enjoyment/energy for sex)?	☐
Staying inactive so that you are far less physically active than before?	☐
If you have a religious faith: have you reduced or stopped reading your Holy book, praying or going to meetings?	☐

From your list and your diary choose a **single** target to change first. This is particularly important if you have ticked several boxes in the checklist. It isn't possible to overcome all these areas at once.

You need to decide on **one** area to concentrate on. Pick an activity that gives you a boost and which also fits with your values/ideals of how you want to live your life.

Choosing a first target

Example: Anne's avoidance

Look back at Anne's example. Anne is doing far less than before. Looking at her diary, she notices several things that give her pleasure, things she values doing and provide a sense of achievement, or that help her feel close to others.

Anne decides that she will make a change by planning to keep up with the housework. She chooses this because when the housework isn't done it upsets her. She has struggled to keep up with it and lies awake at night worrying about how it is so out of hand. This is her first target to add to her activity plan.

Write down the one problem area you want to work on here. (Remember that this should be problem of reduced activity that is worsening how you feel.)

Overcoming Anxiety, Stress and Panic © Dr Chris Williams 2015

Do you need to break your target into smaller steps?

 Example: Anne breaks her target into smaller steps

Anne's target is quite a big problem. There are many things she could do (ironing, vacuuming, dusting, cleaning out cupboards, etc). She looks at the target and feels overwhelmed. So Anne goes through the questions for effective change and decides her target isn't realistic. She breaks it down into smaller tasks. She decides to start by focusing on the ironing.

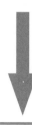

 Q Do you need to break your target down into a number of smaller more achievable targets?

If you answered 'No', go straight to Step 2. If you answered 'Yes', then keep reading about how to choose a realistic first target.

Go back to thinking about your problem. What smaller steps could help you move forward? If you need to, rewrite your first target.

My clear first step is:

Plan the steps needed to carry out your chosen solution

You need to have a clear plan that lays out exactly **what** you are going to do and **when** you are going to do it. This will help you to think about what to do and predict problems that might arise. That way you can think about how you will respond to keep your plan on track if problems arise.

Complete the *Planner sheet* questions to create a good plan.

Your plan

1. What am I going to do?

2. When am I going to do it?

Write in the day and time:

3. Is my planned task one that:

Will be useful for helping me move forward?	Yes ☐	No ☐
Is clear, so that I will know when I have done it?	Yes ☐	No ☐
Is something that I value, or need to do?	Yes ☐	No ☐
Is realistic, practical and achievable?	Yes ☐	No ☐

4. What problems/difficulties could arise, and how can I overcome them?

What could get in the way? Write your possible blocks in here:

Do you need to rewrite your plan to tackle these possible blocks?

5. Write down your final plan here:

What I'm going to do.

When I'm going to do it (day and time).

Remember, if you feel worse with symptoms you can still choose to do the planned activity anyway – because it's important.

Example: Anne's plan

1. **What am I going to do?** Iron in the lounge.
2. **When am I going to do it?** This afternoon at 2.00 p.m. – I know my arthritis is most settled then.
3. **Is my planned task one that:**

Will be useful for helping me move forward?   Yes ☐   No ☐

Is clear, so that I will know when I have done it?   Yes ☐   No ☐

Is something that I value, or need to do?   Yes ☐   No ☐

Is realistic, practical and achievable?   Yes ☐   No ☐

4. **What problems/difficulties could arise, and how can I overcome this?**

There's a power plug in the lounge and an extension wire to plug the iron into. I might feel I have to keep ironing for ages. I'll therefore bring only five items at first. That way I won't feel upset by what's not done. I'll iron for no more than 30 minutes, and not more than 20 items in all. That way I can avoid overly throwing myself into things. I'll also watch my favourite TV programme as I iron.

What might block my plan?

If someone comes to the door I'll need to break off. I'll make sure I tell my sister Mary that I'm going to do some of the ironing and ask her not to pop by until later. Finally, sometimes I know I feel so tired I might not fancy ironing. I have learned that telling someone else what I'm going to do can help keep me motivated to do it – so I'll choose to tell Mary what I plan to do. If I feel tired, I'll choose to do it anyway – because it's important.

Copies of the *Review sheet* are available at the end of this workbook, and can be downloaded free of charge from **www.llttf.com**.

Carry out your plan

Carry out your plan, paying attention to your thoughts about what will happen before, during and after you have completed your plan. Write any thoughts/fears you noticed here:

Try to do your plan anyway. Good luck!

Next, review the outcome using the Review sheet

Example: Did Anne's plan work?

Anne gets everything set up. She manages to iron two shirts, then the phone rings. It's her brother Jake, and she asks him to phone again in the evening. Anne then starts ironing again and watches the TV programme.

She manages to finish the first five items. So she gets another five. She gets through 14 items, and thinks, 'This is great'. She finally manages to finish ironing 18 items before she decides to stop. Anne is pleased she had set things up so she could feel good every five items rather than being annoyed she didn't manage 'the full 20'. She also was pleased because she could enjoy the TV programme while she ironed. She looks at her diary and sees she has scored highly for both pleasure and a sense of having done things that she values and sees as important.

Now write down your review using the structure from the *Review sheet*.

Your review

What did you plan to do?

Did you attempt the task?　　Yes ☐　　　　No ☐

If yes:

● What went well?

● What didn't go so well?

● What have you learned about from what happened?

● How are you going to apply what you have learned?

Write down any helpful lessons or information you have learned from what happened. If things didn't go quite as you hoped, try to learn from what happened.

Copies of the *Review sheet* are available at the end of this workbook, and can be downloaded free of charge from **www.llttf.com**.

What if symptoms get in the way?

It's quite common to find that you might be tempted to put tasks off ("I'll do it tomorrow") or talk yourself out of doing them. You might be feeling worse at the time – perhaps tired, lower in mood, more negative or fed up.

If that's the case, then choose to change what you say to yourself. Instead of saying 'I was going to do it, but feel really tired/stiff/down/fed up/anxious', change it to: 'I'm going to choose to do it even though I feel really tired/stiff/down/fed up/anxious'.

> ### KEY POINT
> The best way of testing out fears and concerns is to act against them and see what happens. If you have planned something that will move you forward, don't let feelings put you off. Even if you feel bad, choose to do it – and see what happens. You may be pleasantly surprised.

Planning the next steps

The next step is to plan another activity to build on your first one. You need to think again about your **short-, medium-** and **longer-term** targets. Did your plan help you completely tackle the activity you were working on? You may need to plan out other solutions to tackle different aspects of your problem. The key is to build one step on another and to start to plan a range of activities across the week and across each day (morning, afternoon and evening). Using the activity sheets to plan these activities can help, so it's clear what you'll do and when.

Each step should be realistic, practical and achievable. Without a step-by-step approach, you may take some steps forward, but they may all be in different directions – and you will lose your focus and motivation. Use what you have just learned to build on what you did.

 ## Example: Anne's short-, medium- and longer-term targets

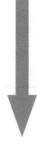

Short term – What might Anne do over the next week or so? This is the next step she needs to plan.
Anne's target: I want to keep working on the ironing until I am up to date with it.

Medium term – What might Anne aim towards doing over the next few weeks – the next few steps?
Anne's target: I want to start going for a walk out of the flat. I used to love going to the park – and it's important to me as a person to keep reasonably fit and to be sociable.

Example: Anne's short-, medium- and longer-term targets (*continued*)

Longer term: Where does Anne want to be in a few months or so?
Anne's target: I need to plan to do things nearly every day. It will help me form more of a routine to my day. I'll keep planning to do this using my Planner sheets. If something comes up and I can't do it on a particular day, I won't beat myself up but just do it the next day.

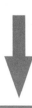

Now it's your turn. In creating your plan:

Do:

- Plan to build activities over the next week.

- Plan to alter things slowly in a step-by-step way.

- Choose activities that help to boost how you feel – those that give you a sense of pleasure and that you value, see as important, or help you feel close to others.

- Include activities you have cut down on or stopped doing but which you know helped how you felt in the past.

- Don't forget to plan activities across the morning, afternoon and evening. Also plan across the week.

- It can be tempting to cut out some key essential activities because it can feel hard to do them. Choose to do some of these tasks each week.

- Remember, if a planned activity is important, it's important to do it even if you feel worse on the day. Choose to do it even if you do feel bad.

- Write down your plan in detail so that you know exactly what you are going to do this week.

Don't:

- Try to alter too many things at once.

- Choose something that is too hard a target to start with.

- Be negative and think 'It's a waste of time'. Try to experiment to find out if this negative thinking is actually valid.

Write your own short-, medium- and long-term plans here:

- **Short term** – What might you do over the next week or so? This is the next step you need to plan.

- **Medium term** – What might you aim towards doing over the next few weeks – the next few steps?

- **Longer term** – Where do you want to be in a few months or so?

Summary

In this workbook you have:

- Learned how low mood and stress cause you to do less.
- Identified things you have cut down or stopped doing which you used to enjoy.
- Started to rebuild a pattern to your day – and planned to tackle key essential tasks.
- Discovered ways to make slow, steady changes to your life to boost how you feel – even if sometimes it feels hard.
- Considered how to live life in a way that fits with your values.
- Planned some next steps to build on these changes.

 What have I learned from this workbook?

What do I want to try *next*?

Getting more help

The course module *I can't be bothered doing anything* has more hints and tips to help you get going. You can work this through at **www.llttf.com**.

Putting into practice what you have learned

You are likely to make the most progress if you can put into practice what you have learned in the workbook.

Suggested reading

The *Noticing extreme and unhelpful thinking* workbook is a good one to read next. Or you can choose to work on another issue that is affecting how you feel.

Plan, Do and Review

Once you have a plan, the next step is to do (or not do) it, and finally to review what has happened. The *Planner sheet* takes care of the planning part. The next step is to use the *Review sheet* to consider how things have gone, good or bad, and learn from it. Copies of both sheets are found at the end of the workbook, and as with all the worksheets can be downloaded from www.llttf.com.

Other sources of support

 www.llttf.com

This popular resource is designed to support readers of this course. There's also a forum where you can make comments, or ask questions of other people using the same course.

Acknowledgments

The cartoon illustrations were produced by Keith Chan, kchan75@hotmail.com.

The terms LLTTF and Five Areas are registered trademarks of Five Areas Resources Ltd.

Although we hope you find this book helpful, it's not intended to be a direct substitute for consultative advice with a healthcare professional, nor do we give any assurance about its effectiveness in a particular case. Accordingly, neither the publisher nor the author shall be held liable for any loss or damages arising from its use.

Planner sheet

My plan to take things forward:

1. *What* am I going to do?

2. *When* am I going to do it?

Write in the day and time:

3. Is my planned task one that:

		Yes	No
Q Will be useful for helping me move forward?		Yes ☐	No ☐
Q Is clear, so that I will know when I have done it?		Yes ☐	No ☐
Q Is something that I value, or need to do?		Yes ☐	No ☐
Q Is realistic, practical and achievable?		Yes ☐	No ☐

4. What problems/difficulties could arise, and how can I overcome this?

What could get in the way? Write your possible blocks in here:

Do you need to rewrite your plan to tackle these possible blocks?

5. Write down your final plan here

What I'm going to do.

When I'm going to do it (day and time).

KEY POINT

If you feel worse with symptoms you can still choose to do the planned activity anyway – because it's important.

Review sheet

What did you plan to do?

Write it here.

Did you attempt the task?   Yes ☐   No ☐

If yes:

● What went well?

● What didn't go so well?

● What have you learned about from what happened?

● How are you going to apply what you have learned?

If not:

What stopped you?

● *Internal factors* (forgot, not enough time, put it off, concerns I couldn't do it, I couldn't see the point of it, etc.)

● *External factors* (events that happened, work/home issues, etc.)

● How could you have planned to tackle these blocks?

Use the *Plan, Do, Review* approach to help you move forward.

My activity (activities across the day and week)

Date and time	Activity (include everything you do)	Duration How long did you do it for?	Pleasure felt 0= No pleasure 10= maximum pleasure	What is the value/importance to you of the activity? 0= Not important at all 10= maximum importance	Sense of closeness to others 0= No sense of closeness 10= maximum sense of closeness
Morning					
Afternoon					
Evening					

Worksheets to help you practice *Doing things that boost how you feel*

Practice is important to help you master this approach. You can download worksheets of all of the key skills used in this workbook from:
www.llttf.com/worksheets/odlm

My notes

Using exercise to boost how you feel

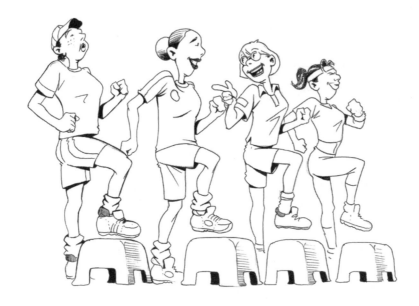

www.llttf.com or www.livinglifetothefull.com ⒠ @llttfnews (public)

www.fiveareas.com ⒠ @fiveareas (practitioners)

⨍ www.llttf.com/facebook

Dr Chris Williams

overcoming
depression and low mood
a five areas approach

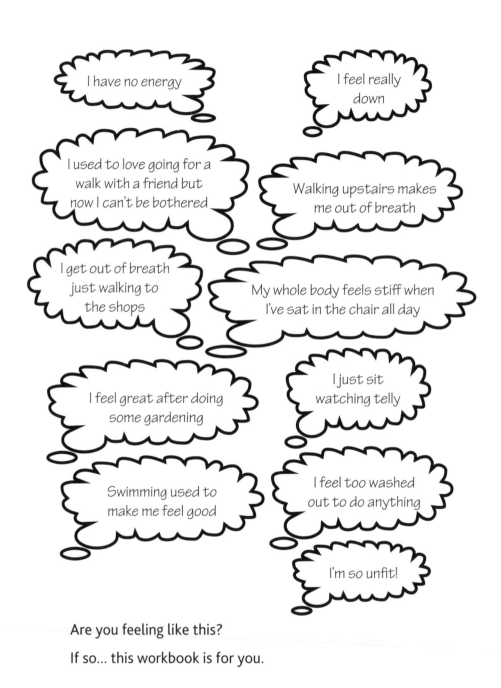

Are you feeling like this?

If so... this workbook is for you.

Why bother with exercise?

Think about a time when you had a bad cold. Besides a runny nose and a sore throat – did you feel subdued, fed up and down emotionally as well?

Now think back to a time when you exercised – such as riding a bike, running or swimming. Some people find that they feel happier and calmer after exercise.

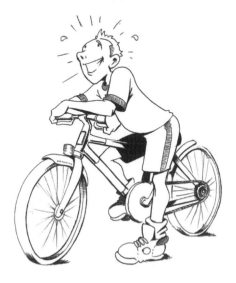

Your emotions, your thinking, your behaviour, your relationships, your life situation and your body all affect each other. Look at the five areas diagram.

Each of the five areas is connected. That's why by **increasing your physical activity levels, you can boost how you feel** mentally as well as physically.

In this workbook you will:

- See how exercise can boost your mood.
- Learn how to use exercise to reduce your tension and anxiety.
- Discover how exercise can help you feel more fit and better about yourself.

The benefits of exercise

People often forget to exercise when they feel unwell, or it just seems too hard to do. Exercise can be 'prescribed' by doctors as part of treatment for depression. But you can also choose to 'prescribe' it to yourself as part of your own self-treatment plan.

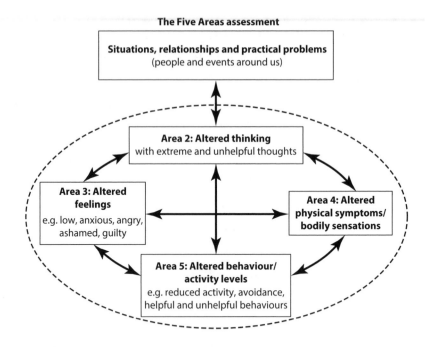

The Five Areas assessment

Exercise can be fun if you choose something that you previously enjoyed doing.

It gives you control so you can plan things at your own pace.

It can help you structure and plan your day – rather than staying in and being inactive.

It can boost your social life. Doing things with others such as a step class, playing football or going for a swim can help you meet other people with a shared interest.

Even with a baby you can exercise. Check out whether there are any aqua-aerobics or mother/baby exercise or massage classes in your area.

If you have a baby or toddler, walking with the pram (and another mum) is also good exercise.

It really is a win-win situation.

Are there any reasons not to exercise?

- If you are physically unwell, you may not be able to do certain exercises. Ask your doctor or health visitor for advice about what you can or can't do if you are ill or have had a recent operation.

- You may have aching muscles to begin with (the author does). Make sure you pace things.

- There can be a cost for some activities (for example, for using a gym or a swimming pool).

KEY POINT

Exercise and injury: Remember it's important to **warm up to avoid muscle pulls, aches and strains**. Using good techniques and the right equipment, clothing and shoes is also important.

How planned exercise can help you feel better

Experiment

You'll need less than 15 minutes to do this experiment. The aim is to test if even a small amount of exercise affects how you feel overall.

Before you start, think of a physical activity that you can do. This should be something:

- That is realistic, bearing in mind your current physical condition.

- That can be done in just 5 to 10 minutes to start with.

- You know is within your capabilities and doesn't push you.

Please choose something just now that doesn't involve vigorous exercise. For example, walk up and down a flight of stairs three to four times. Take a rest if you get out of breath.

KEY POINT

The above experiment is not a full workout. You don't need to change into gym gear, work up a sweat or even do warm-up exercises!

Other things you could try are stretching, jogging slowly in one spot or walking round the block at a reasonable pace. If you have a small child, you can do the last one with your child in a pram. Remember not to overdo it.

Aim to do something that gets your heart rate up and gets you moving **without being excessive**. Remember, the benefits can be boosted even more by doing activities that are fun or sociable. If you are physically unwell you should always check what is appropriate with your doctor first.

Doing your planned exercise

So you've chosen what to do. **Before you start** mark the two charts below to show how you feel right now.

How you feel before your exercise

Now do your 5 to 10 minutes of exercise. Remember you can stop for a rest if you are getting tired.

Your review

Immediately afterwards please rate your mood again.

How you feel after your exercise

Next: stop, think and reflect

Have a look at your scores before and after.

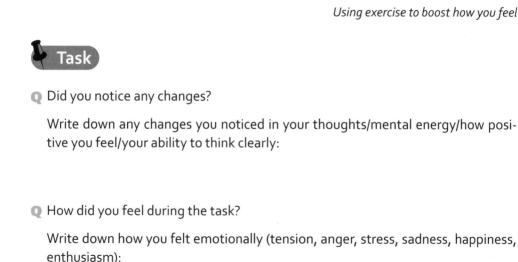

Task

Q Did you notice any changes?

Write down any changes you noticed in your thoughts/mental energy/how positive you feel/your ability to think clearly:

Q How did you feel during the task?

Write down how you felt emotionally (tension, anger, stress, sadness, happiness, enthusiasm):

Q How did you feel physically?

Write down here how you felt physically (relaxed/tense, jittery, tired, achy, ready for more):

Write down any other changes you noticed:

Q Overall, do you think you might benefit from planning some exercise into your life as part of your own 'mental fitness' package?

Yes ☐   No ☐   Yes, but… ☐

Yes, but …

There are lots of things in life that we know are good for us, but we don't do them. Remember, that's just as true in other people's lives as it may be in your own.

Tackling the simple blocks

Often the biggest problems are simple ones:

- Perhaps you just aren't in the habit of doing exercise.
- Or maybe you want to get into the habit of doing exercise but you think it will be too hard. It's easy to talk yourself out of it or say there's no time.

Many people see exercise as too hard or boring, too expensive, taking too much time – or all of these!

 What thoughts block you from doing exercise? Write them down here:

Planning to do exercise doesn't mean you have to make a big change to your lifestyle. Even **small changes** can make a positive difference.

Making a clear plan that works for you

People are often amazed at how empowering, energizing and good it can feel when they get into the habit of exercising as part of their regular daily routine.

- Choose something that speeds up your heart rate and breathing at least a little. Be sensible based on your physical health.

- Build up the amount of exercise slowly and gradually; plan increases in increments.

- Don't throw yourself into things too quickly (or start too slowly): **pacing is the key**.

- Many people find that doing exercise at the start of the day gives them energy for the day. Try to avoid exercising just before going to bed as this can unhelpfully affect your sleep.

- Plan to exercise with a friend or relative. This has the added benefit of encouraging you to go when you don't feel like it. It will also help boost your **sense of closeness**, which again will help your mood.

- Walking with your children or partner or a friend, talking about what you see as you walk or just having general conversation, is a good example of cheap and effective exercise.

- If you are married or have a partner, sex can be a great way of being active, using calories, building your relationship and aiding sleep.

- If you've signed up for the **www.llttf.com/www.livinglifetothefull.com** course you can request short **e-mail reminders** to help keep you on track. These are free and you can cancel at any time. (Please note the course doesn't offer advice on an individual basis.)

Planning when and how to exercise

Exercising on a regular basis – even if it is just a short time to begin with – is important. It is best to plan this into your day and diary rather than just 'trying to fit it in sometime'. You may find the following **planning task** helpful in making this regular commitment.

My plan to use exercise to help me feel better

What am I going to do?

Remember to choose something that is possible, realistic and achievable. Preferably something that is fun. Think about planning some exercise that has a social aspect at least once a week – for example walking with a friend, a step or yoga class or going for a run or walk with others. Exercise doesn't need to cost lots of money. You can get exercise videos and DVDs from your local library and many examples are available to watch for free online. Or you could walk to your local shop each time you need something instead of taking the bus or driving.

Write your target here:

When am I going to do it?

Decide whether doing some exercise every day is practical for you. If it is, what time of day would be best for you? If you can't manage it every day, then how about just once or twice a week? You can always build upon this at a later stage.

Write in the day and time:

Is my planned task one that:

Will be useful for helping me move forward?	Yes ☐	No ☐
Is clear, so that I will know when I have done it?	Yes ☐	No ☐
Is something that I value, or need to do?	Yes ☐	No ☐
Is realistic, practical and achievable?	Yes ☐	No ☐

What problems/difficulties could arise, and how can I overcome this? What could get in the way? For example your daily routine, work or family deadlines such as picking up children from school, money, or having the sports equipment or clothing you need. Be realistic – think about your current level of fitness, health and motivation. If you have doubts about your health, please discuss this with your doctor.

Write your possible blocks in here:

Do you need to rewrite your plan to tackle these possible blocks?

Write down your final plan here.

What are you going to do?

When are you going to do it? (day and time)

Your back-up plan: Think of another back-up solution you could turn to if for whatever reason there are problems with your plan.

Keeping on track

Once you have created your exercise plan it is **important to keep on track**. This means setting yourself short-, medium- and longer-term goals and reviewing your progress. In this way you can make changes if things aren't going well.

My plan for the next few weeks

Think about changes you want to make:

- In the short term (where you want to be in a few weeks' time).

- In the medium term (where you want to be in a few months' time).

- In the long term (where you want to be in a year's time).

Summary
In this workbook you have learned:

- How exercise can boost how you feel.
- The benefits and 'side effects' of exercise.
- Ways of planning exercise into your life in a paced way.

Before you go

 What have you learned from this workbook?

 What do you want to try *next*?

Putting into practice what you have learned

Here are some more ideas to help you as you plan to increase your exercise regime:

- Your doctor/physician may be able to refer you to an exercise class you can attend free of charge.

- Look out for classes at your local swimming pool or gym. Some pools and gyms also have crèches or children's clubs for babies or children.

- Think about tennis, badminton or walking classes.

- Do exercise with a friend or colleague.

Plan, Do and Review

Whatever you choose to do, the first step is to make a plan and then try it out. The *Planner sheet* will help you create a clear and realistic plan. The next step is to use the *Review sheet* to consider how things have gone – and whether good or bad to learn from it. Copies of both sheets are found at the end of the workbook, and as with all the worksheets can be downloaded from www.llttf.com. Try to establish a routine of *Plan, Do* and *Review*.

Other sources of support

 www.llttf.com (www.livinglifetothefull.com; @llttfnews**)**

This popular resource is designed to support readers of this course. There's also a forum where you can make comments, or ask questions of other people using the same course.

Acknowledgments

The cartoon illustrations were produced by Keith Chan, kchan75@hotmail.com.

The terms LLTTF and Five Areas are registered trademarks of Five Areas Resources Ltd.

Although we hope you find this book helpful, it's not intended to be a direct substitute for consultative advice with a healthcare professional, nor do we give any assurance about its effectiveness in a particular case. Accordingly, neither the publisher nor the author shall be held liable for any loss or damages arising from its use.

Planner sheet

1. *What* am I going to do?

2. *When* am I going to do it?

Write in the day and time:

3. Is my planned task one that:

Q Will be useful for helping me move forward?	Yes ☐	No ☐
Q Is clear, so that I will know when I have done it?	Yes ☐	No ☐
Q Is something that I value, or need to do?	Yes ☐	No ☐
Q Is realistic, practical and achievable?	Yes ☐	No ☐

4. What problems/difficulties could arise, and how can I overcome these?

What could get in the way? Write your possible blocks in here:

Do you need to rewrite your plan to tackle these possible blocks?

5. Write down your final plan here

What are you going to do?

When are you going to do it? (day and time)

Your back-up plan: Think of another back-up solution you could turn to if for whatever reason there are problems with your plan.

KEY POINT
If you feel worse you can choose to do the planned activity anyway – because it's important.

Review sheet

What did you plan to do?

Write it here.

What happened? Did you attempt the task? Yes ☐ No ☐

If yes:

● What went well?

● What didn't go so well?

● What have you learned about from what happened?

● How are you going to apply what you've learned?

If not:

What stopped you?

● *Internal factors* (e.g. forgot, not enough time, put it off, concerns I couldn't do it, I couldn't see the point of it, etc.)

● *External factors* (events that happened, work/home issues, etc.)

● How could you have planned to tackle these blocks?

Use the *Plan, Do, Review* approach to help you move forward.

Overcoming Anxiety, Stress and Panic © Dr Chris Williams 2015

Worksheets to help you practice *Using exercise to boost how you feel*

Practice is important to help you master this approach. You can download worksheets of all of the key skills used in this workbook from:
www.llttf.com/worksheets/odlm

My notes

Helpful things you can do

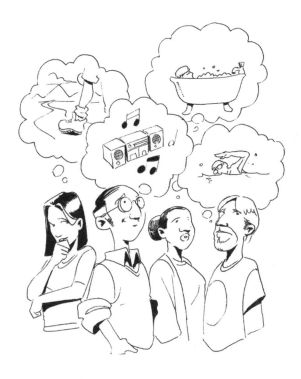

www.llttf.com or www.livinglifetothefull.com 🅑 @llttfnews (public)

www.fiveareas.com 🅑 @fiveareas (practitioners)

f www.llttf.com/facebook

Dr Chris Williams

overcoming
depression and low mood
a five areas approach

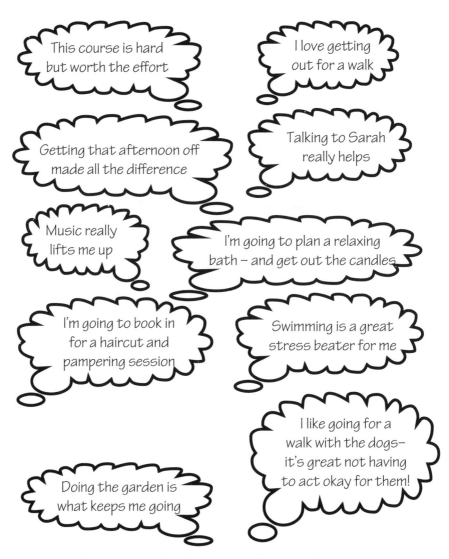

Are you doing things that boost you, like these?

If not... this workbook is for you.

Overcoming Anxiety, Stress and Panic © Dr Chris Williams 2015

In this workbook you will:

- Learn about helpful things you can do that can give you a boost.
- Plan some ways to make sure that you do these things, even when you are busy.

What are helpful activities?

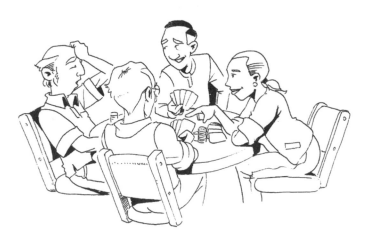

Helpful activities include:

- Talking to or meeting up with family or friends.

- Doing things that give you a boost, for example getting outside, walking in the park, reading a book or going swimming –things that often fall by the wayside when you begin to feel down.

- Pampering yourself, such as having a special bath with music and candles, or a nice meal, a haircut or something else you enjoy. It doesn't have to be costly.

- Seeking accurate information about how to tackle low mood and depression. For example, reading books like this one, or reading information leaflets and fact sheets that you can get from charities and other major organizations that support people with depression. A list of these is available online at **www.llttf.com**.

- Seeing your doctor to find out what support is available for you locally; for example, an expert mental health worker.

- Keeping going – activity helps overcome low mood. Get outside, and say hello to people you know as you go for a walk. Things like this will boost your confidence.

Task

Write down any *helpful* things you have done in the past two weeks.

It makes sense to actively plan these things into your week. In this way you will give yourself little boosts throughout the week.

Helpful activities serve the following purposes:

● They boost how you feel

● They help in the short **and** longer term

● They help how you and others around you feel

Building helpful habits into your life is an important way of feeling better.

The impact of helpful behaviours on you

Think about any behaviours you do that help you.

 What effect do they have on you and those around you, in the short and longer term?
Choose just one recent example and write down how it helps.

Effect on me

Consider the impact on each of five key areas of your life:

Altered thinking: Did it give you a positive view of the situation, of you or others? Were you living according to your values/ideals?

Altered feelings/emotions: Did it make you feel happy/content?

Altered physical symptoms/bodily sensations: Was the behaviour good for your body?

Altered behaviour: Did it help you develop any helpful habits of responding?

Effect on others

Helpful behaviours are often good both for you and also others.

What is the impact on others around you? Was your behaviour helpful for them also?

So there are all sorts of good reasons to plan to build in more helpful responses to your day and week. But how can you plan to do this?

Have a clear plan

You will need to decide:

- **Short-term** targets – changes you can make today, tomorrow and next week.
- **Medium-term** targets – changes over the next few weeks.
- **Long-term** targets – where you want to be in six months or a year.

That way you can build positive changes step by step.

When helpful things can become unhelpful

Sometimes you may think that an activity is helpful, but in fact it's part of the problem. For example:

- Drinking a lot to settle your nerves or provide false confidence
- Avoiding people and events around you that make you feel stressed
- Seeking reassurance – like an addiction, you keep needing more

KEY POINT
Many helpful things you do can become unhelpful for you or for others if you rely on them too much or do them all the time.

Now let's move on to possible ways in which you can build helpful behaviours into your life.

Building helpful responses

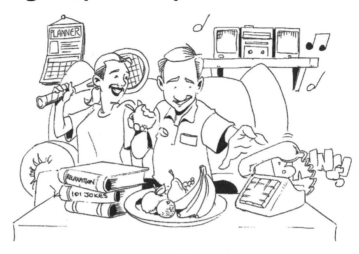

Some activities may seem quite easy to do right away. Others may need some planning using the seven-step plan below.

Step 1: Identify and clearly define what you will work on

The first thing to do is to choose a single helpful behaviour to work on first.

Look at the following list and tick any activity that you used to do, but have cut down or stopped because of how you feel.

What helpful things have you cut down or stopped?

Are you:	Tick here if you have cut down or stopped doing this
Being good to yourself? For example, eating regularly and healthily, taking time to enjoy the food.	☐
Doing things for fun/pleasure? For example, your hobbies, listening to music, having a nice bath.	☐

Overcoming Anxiety, Stress and Panic © Dr Chris Williams 2015

Seeking support from others whom you trust? Like going to a self-help group meeting (your GP can tell you about these groups).	☐
Keeping in touch with others even if you don't feel like it? Pick a level of contact you can cope with, for example by telephone, e-mail or meeting up.	☐
Stopping, thinking and reflecting on things rather than jumping to conclusions? For example, letting upsetting thoughts 'just be' rather than ruminating on them.	☐
Finding out accurate information about depression by reading information leaflets, self-help books, etc?	☐
Pacing yourself – so as not to run out of energy or sit doing very little?	☐
Keeping active physically? For example, doing exercise/going for walks/swimming/gardening/riding your bike. *Note:* If you have had an operation or are physically ill and in pain, you may need to take it easy for a time. But once your doctor says it's okay, try to keep reasonably active. If you rest too much you will find you feel stiffer and more easily tired. Try walking with as relaxed and normal a posture as possible.	☐
Using your sense of humour to cope?	☐
Giving yourself a break/the benefit of the doubt? Remember: No-one is perfect.	☐
Taking any prescribed medication regularly and/or as prescribed? Remember that the medication is there to help.	☐
Using approaches such as relaxation tapes, slow breathing, etc. to deal with tension? (See www.llttf.com/www.livinglifetothefull.)	☐

(Continued)

Being honest with trusted others (especially your GP) about how you really are? If you are struggling, you need to say so, otherwise people will not know you need help.	☐
If you have children: Planning time for yourself, or you and your partner together without the children? You could plan to leave your baby with a friend, relative or in a crèche while you spend time together talking or doing adult things like going out for a meal.	☐
If you have children: Playing with your children and spending time together reading stories or having cuddles?	☐

List any other helpful behaviours you do here:

Next, use this checklist to choose a target to work on first.

Example: Julia's target

Julia has been feeling depressed for a second time in her life. Her son Ben is 11 years old and it's the summer holidays. Julia has felt increasingly ground down by her low mood and has been doing less and less for herself. She knows that meeting up with others gives her a boost. Julia completes the checklist and decides she will plan some time with her friends.

Now it's your turn

Look back at your responses and choose **one** behaviour that you focus on building first. This is particularly important if you have ticked many boxes in the list. It isn't possible to do everything at once, so you need to decide which **one** area to focus on to start with.

My target: Write down a single helpful behaviour that you want to work on:

KEY POINT
Remember that this should be a helpful behaviour that has helped you before, but which you have stopped or cut down doing. Choose an activity that you would like to do. You can choose any, but it's often helpful to choose things you know from previous experience will help you.

Breaking it down into smaller steps

The important thing is to use a **step-by-step** approach so that no single step seems too large. The first step should be something that gets you moving in the right direction. For instance, to go to the cinema with friends you might need to decide who to ask, check what films are playing, decide which film to go to, how to get there and back, etc. You can plan all of these stages with a step-by-step approach. Once you've picked the first step to work on, move on to Step 2.

Step 2: Think up as many ways as possible to achieve your first target

Consider ways to work out how to do the activity. If you hit a dead end, step back from the problem and try to think of other solutions. This approach is called **brainstorming**. The more solutions that you can think of, the more likely it is that a good one will emerge. The purpose of brainstorming is to try to come up with **as many ideas as possible**, and from there it will be easier for you to identify a good solution.

KEY POINT
You can include ridiculous ideas at first to get yourself to start thinking more flexibly!

Example: Julia's ideas

- First a crazy idea – I could fly everyone out to a desert island!
- I could invite some friends for lunch.
- I could invite one or two friends for a walk in the park.
- I could do something with others and leave my son Ben with some-one, like mum.
- I could invite all my friends round for a party in the evening when Ben is in bed.
- I could watch a film with a friend.

To help you come up with a list of possible solutions, think about these things:

Q What advice would you give a friend who was trying to make the same changes? Sometimes it's easier to think of solutions for others than for ourselves.

Q What *ridiculous* solutions can you include as well as sensible ones?

Q What helpful ideas would others (e.g. family, friends or colleagues) suggest?

Q What have you tried in the past that was helpful?

> **KEY POINT**
> If you feel stuck, sometimes doing this task with someone you trust can be helpful.

Step 3: Look at the pros and cons of each possible activity

 Example: Looking at Julia's ideas

Ideas from step 2	Pros	Cons
First a crazy idea – I could fly everyone out to a desert island!	It would be nice. Maybe we could have an all-inclusive holiday with a youth club.	There isn't the money at the moment. That's one of those whacky ideas to start off with!
I could invite some friends for lunch.	That would be fun. It would be nice to see some friends and Ben could join us at the table.	I know what I'm like – I'd worry about the cooking if it was a big meal – so it would need to be small and easy to prepare.

(Continued)

Overcoming Anxiety, Stress and Panic © Dr Chris Williams 2015

Example: Looking at Julia's ideas *(Continued)*

Ideas from step 2	Pros	Cons
I could invite one or two friends for a walk in the park.	Getting out might be good fun.	What if it rained? What would Ben do – he hates walks in the park?
I could do something with others and leave Ben with someone, like mum.	I'd have some free time – and could chat and enjoy time with others.	Mum is pretty busy herself. I'd have to make sure she was okay about this and not stay away too long.
I could invite all my friends round for a party in the evening when Ben is in bed.	It would be good to chat to the adults.	I'm not sure – it's a lot for me to arrange on my own.
I could go see a film with a friend.	I used to like going to films and haven't been out anywhere for a long time. I'd love to see that new romantic comedy.	I couldn't take Ben. Might someone be able to look after him for two to three hours?

Write down your list of possible helpful activities into the following table, along with the pros and cons of each suggestion.

My suggestions from Step 2	Pros (advantages)	Cons (disadvantages)

Step 4: Choose one of the activities

From your list in Step 3, pick an activity that is realistic and likely to give you a boost. Choose something that gets you moving in the right direction. This should be small enough to be possible, but big enough to move you forward. It can be helpful to think of this as one of many small steps that will help you move forward.

Example: Julia's first step

Julia decides to ask her friends Jamila and Andrea round for lunch (her second idea). Jamila's son, Imran, is in the same year as Ben. She knows they get on well and will play together.

Look at your own responses in Step 3 and then choose what you will do.

My choice

Write down your preferred option here:

Check your choice

Now see if you can answer 'Yes' to the questions below.

Is my planned solution one that:

Q Will be useful for helping me move forward?   Yes ☐   No ☐

Q Is clear, so that I will know when I have done it?   Yes ☐   No ☐

Q Is something that I value, or need to do?   Yes ☐   No ☐

Q Is realistic, practical and achievable?   Yes ☐   No ☐

If you answered 'Yes' to all four questions, the step you chose is a good one to start with. If you answered 'No', then think again and choose another option from your list.

Step 5: Plan the steps needed for your chosen solution

You need to have a clear plan that lays out exactly **what** you are going to do and **when** you are going to do it. *Write down* the steps needed to carry out your plan. Use the *Planner sheet* at the end of this workbook to help you do this.

This will help you to think about what to do and to predict possible problems that might arise. Remember that an important part of the planning process is to predict what might block the plan. That way you can think about how you will respond to keep your plan on track if there are problems.

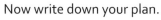

Example: Julia's plan

What are you going to do?

Julia phones her two friends Jamila and Andrea. They have a nice catch-up on the phone.

When are you going to do it?

They agree that they will meet next Tuesday for lunch at Julia's house and then go for a walk in the park if the weather's nice.

Julia decides that to make the visit less stressful she will make the food easy – heat some pizzas and have some salad.

What problems or difficulties could arise?

She tries to think of anything that might block the plan or cause problems. She predicts that Ben will keep popping in wanting things, and that could be stressful.

She also wonders what would happen if one of her friends gets ill and can't come?

How could you overcome these difficulties?

She tells Ben beforehand that she wants some time with her friends, and encourages him to think about playing football outside at the park with Jamila's son Imran.

She thinks through what she will do if someone is ill or cannot come. She will phone round and if this happens, they'd try to plan lunch or perhaps watching a film together at some other time.

Now write down your plan.

 What are you going to do?

 When are you going to do it?

What problems or difficulties could arise?

 How could you overcome them?

Choose a back-up plan

It's good to have a back-up solution for if difficulties arise with your first choice plan.

Example: Julia's Julia's back-up plan

Julia decides that if her first plan doesn't work, she will plan to invite a friend round to watch a film.

Write your own back-up plan here:

Step 6: Carry out the plan

Your task is to carry out this plan during the next week. Here's where you find out if all that planning has helped.

Example 1: Julia tries her plan

Julia buys the pizza and salad the day before her get-together from the local shop. On the day of the get-together Andrea phones to say her mum is sick and she can't come. Julia is about to burst into tears and is tempted to phone Jamila and cancel but she decides that she will go ahead with the plan with Jamila anyway.

Jamila and Imran come round. Julia and Jamila have a nice meal with the boys, and then they chat while Ben and Imran play football in the park. Julia is happy and feels a sense of achievement, and also a real sense of closeness to her friend. She and Jamila then go to the park and chat with the boys, and then continue their walk together. They agree to meet again at Jamila's house the next week and will see if Andrea can join them then.

Overcoming Anxiety, Stress and Panic © Dr Chris Williams 2015

Pay attention to any thoughts and fears about what will happen before, during and after you have completed your plan. Write any thoughts/fears you noticed here:

Try to carry out your plan anyway.

Step 7: Review the outcome

Whatever happened, now is the time to review the plan and learn from your experience.

 Example: Julia reviews her plan

> The lunch was great. It would have been so easy for me to cancel. When Andrea called off I was really upset. I'm glad I didn't call it off, though, because Jamila and I had a great time. It really made me feel good. I know Jamila enjoyed it too – and we hope to meet up with Andrea at her place next week. It's also great that Imran and Ben played so well. They've arranged to meet again tomorrow to play some more football. That will be great for me too!
>
> I'm looking forward to next week.

Review what happened with the *Review sheet* (copies of which are at the end of this workbook). You can answer the same questions below.

What did you plan to do?

What happened? Did you attempt the task?　　　　　　Yes ☐　　　No ☐

If yes:

● What went well?

● What didn't go so well?

- What have you learned about from what happened?

- How are you going to apply what you've learned?

If not:

What stopped you?

- *Internal factors* (e.g. forgot, not enough time, put it off, concerns I couldn't do it, I couldn't see the point of it, etc.)

- *External factors* (events that happened, work/home issues, etc.)

- How could you have planned to tackle these blocks?

Use the *Plan, Do, Review* approach to help you move forward.

If you noticed problems with your plan

Choosing realistic targets for change is important. Think back to where you started – were you too ambitious or unrealistic in choosing the target you did? Sometimes your attempt to solve a problem may be blocked by something unexpected. Perhaps something didn't happen as you planned, or someone reacted in an unexpected way? Try to learn from what happened.

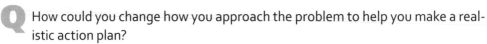 How could you change how you approach the problem to help you make a realistic action plan?

Planning the next steps

Now that you have reviewed how your first step went, the next step is to plan another helpful change to build on this first one. You need to think about your **short-, medium-** and **longer-term** targets. This means where you want to be in a few weeks' time (short term), in a few months' time (medium term) or in a year's time (long term).

> **KEY POINT**
> You will need to slowly build on what you have done step-by-step.

You can choose to:

- Repeat the same thing you have just completed.

- Move it on a bit more.

- Practice another helpful behaviour.

Remember to think about the pros and cons of each choice.

Tips for choosing the next helpful behaviour

Create your own clear plan that will move things forward one step at a time.

Do:

- Be realistic. Plan to try **only** one or two activities over the next week.

- Make sure your **plan** includes breaking down your chosen activity into smaller steps if it doesn't seem realistic and practical to do all together.

- Write down your plan in detail so you have a clear idea of what you will do and have predicted things that may block your plan from happening.

Don't:

- Try to plan too big an activity all at once.

- Be negative and think, 'I can't do anything, what's the point, it's a waste of time'. Experiment to find out if this negative thinking is right or helpful.

Write your own short-, medium- and long-term plans here:

- **Short term** – What might you do over the next week or so? This is your next step that you need to plan.

- **Medium term** – What might you aim toward doing over the next few weeks – the next few steps?

- **Longer term** – Where do you want to be in a few months or so?

Remember to plan slow, steady changes. By breaking down problems and tackling them one step at a time any problem can be addressed. Use the *Planner sheet* and *Review sheet* to help you get into a system of *Plan, Do and Review*. Copies of both sheets are found at the end of the workbook, and as with all the worksheets can be downloaded from www.llttf.com.

KEY POINT
Stick to a plan, learn from what happens and make changes step-by-step. You will grow in confidence and find you can slowly build helpful habits into your life.

Summary

In this workbook you have:

- Learned about helpful things you can do that will give you a boost.
- Tried a way of planning that works well to build helpful activities into your life.

Before you go

 What have you learned from this workbook?

 What do you want to try *next*?

Putting into practice what you have learned

You are likely to make the most progress if you can put into practice what you have learned in the workbook.

Continue to put into practice what you learn over the next few weeks. Don't try to tackle every problem behaviour at once. Plan out what to do at a pace that's right for you. Build changes one step at a time. Some problems such as drinking, gambling and others may take lots of time to change direction because they are addictive.

> **KEY POINT**
> Be prepared for setbacks and times when you slip back into the problem after a period of improvement. Don't get stuck in self-criticism. Instead, pick yourself up, dust yourself down and keep planning. Don't put off asking for help if you are stuck.

Plan, Do and Review

Whatever you choose to do, the first step is to make a plan and then try it out. The *Planner sheet* will help you create a clear and realistic plan. The next step is to use the *Review sheet* on page 199 at the end of this workbook to consider how things have gone, and whether good or bad to learn from it. Copies of both sheets are found at the end of the workbook, and as with all the worksheets can be downloaded from www.llttf.com.

Other sources of support

 www.llttf.com (www.livinglifetothefull.com; @llttfnews)

This popular resource is designed to support readers of this course. There's also a forum where you can make comments, or ask questions of other people using the same course.

Acknowledgments

The cartoon illustrations were produced by Keith Chan, kchan75@hotmail.com.

The terms LLTTF and Five Areas are registered trademarks of Five Areas Resources Ltd.

Although we hope you find this book helpful, it's not intended to be a direct substitute for consultative advice with a healthcare professional, nor do we give any assurance about its effectiveness in a particular case. Accordingly, neither the publisher nor the author shall be held liable for any loss or damages arising from its use.

7-Step problem-solving worksheet

Step 1: Identify and clearly define what you will work on

● Select what you are going to work on (your target). Write it down on a separate sheet of paper.

● Is it a large or complex problem? Do you need to break it down into smaller steps? If yes, write down your new target on the sheet of paper.

Step 2: Think up as many solutions as possible to achieve your first target

For this step you will need to **brainstorm** possible solutions. Include ridiculous ideas as well as sensible ones. What would you advise a friend? What advice would others who you respect suggest? Write down all your solutions as you think of them on your sheet of paper.

Step 3: Look at the pros and cons of each possible solution

Write down a list of the pluses and minuses of each option on your sheet of paper. You can draw a table like the one earlier the workbook.

Step 4: Now choose one of the solutions

Use your answers in Step 3 to make this choice. Write this down on your paper under the heading '*My solution*'.

Check if your solution will be:

Useful for helping me move forward	Yes ☐	No ☐
Clear, so that I will know when I have done it	Yes ☐	No ☐
Something that I value, or need to do	Yes ☐	No ☐
Realistic, practical and achievable	Yes ☐	No ☐

Step 5: Plan the steps needed to carry out your chosen solution

Now, write your plan out using the *Planner sheet* at the end of this workbook. Include a back-up plan of what you will do if your solution **doesn't fully work out**.

Step 6: Carry out your plan

Step 7: Review the outcome

Use the *Review sheet* at the end of this workbook. Even if the plan wasn't completely successful, there will be things you will have learned. How can you put what you have learned into practice?

Planner sheet

1. *What* am I going to do?

2. *When* am I going to do it?

Write in the day and time:

3. Is my planned task one that:

Q Will be useful for helping me move forward?	Yes ☐	No ☐
Q Is clear, so that I will know when I have done it?	Yes ☐	No ☐
Q Is something that I value, or need to do?	Yes ☐	No ☐
Q Is realistic, practical and achievable?	Yes ☐	No ☐

4. What problems/difficulties could arise, and how can I overcome these?

What could get in the way? Write your possible blocks in here:

Do you need to rewrite your plan to tackle these possible blocks?

5. Write down your final plan here

What are you going to do?

When are you going to do it? (day and time)

Your back-up plan: Think of another back-up solution you could turn to if for whatever reason there are problems with your plan.

Review sheet

What did you plan to do?

Write it here.

What happened? Did you attempt the task?   Yes ☐   No ☐

If yes:

● What went well?

● What didn't go so well?

● What have you learned about from what happened?

● How are you going to apply what you've learned?

If not:

What stopped you?

● *Internal factors* (e.g. forgot, not enough time, put it off, concerns I couldn't do it, I couldn't see the point of it, etc.)

● *External factors* (events that happened, work/home issues, etc.)

● How could you have planned to tackle these blocks?

Use the *Plan, Do, Review* approach to help you move forward.

Worksheets to help you practice *Helpful things you can do*

Practice is important to help you master this approach. You can download worksheets of all of the key skills used in this workbook from:
www.llttf.com/worksheets/odlm

My notes

Unhelpful things you do

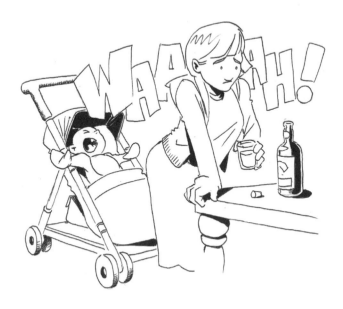

www.llttf.com or www.livinglifetothefull.com @llttfnews (public)

www.fiveareas.com @fiveareas (practitioners)

www.llttf.com/facebook

Dr Chris Williams

overcoming
depression and low mood
a five areas approach

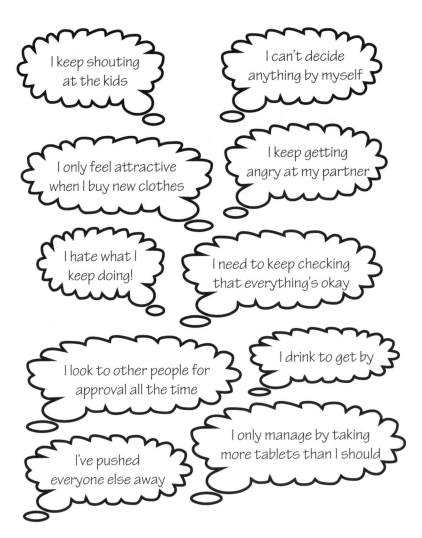

Are you doing things like these?

If so... this workbook is for you.

Overcoming Anxiety, Stress and Panic © Dr Chris Williams 2015

In this workbook you will:

- Find out about how some things can make you feel worse.
- Learn some helpful ways to tackle unhelpful behaviours.
- Make a clear plan to reduce an unhelpful behaviour.
- Plan some next steps to build on this.

Helpful and unhelpful behaviours

When somebody feels distressed, it is normal to try to do things to feel better. But their responses may be *helpful* or *unhelpful*. You can find out more about helpful behaviours in the workbook *Helpful things you can do*.

Unhelpful behaviours

Some examples of common unhelpful behaviours are:

- Getting angry at others.
- Pushing people away.
- Drinking too much to block how you feel.
- Doing things that go against your values/ideals and how you want to live your life.

These behaviours are unhelpful because of the effect they have on everyone. So, getting angry can end up with you feeling alone. This can prevent you getting the help and support the other person would otherwise have offered. So both you and the other person feel worse as a result.

These unhelpful behaviours come in Area 5 of the five areas assessment – Altered behaviours/activity levels. What we do (or don't do) can affect each of the other areas and worsen how we feel. The aim of this workbook is to help you understand why this pattern happens, and also to learn ways of changing that behaviour around.

Why do unhelpful behaviours happen?

People tend to do unhelpful things simply because these actions can make them feel better – **in the short term**. So an activity like getting drunk might be fun, gambling or fighting might be exciting – for a time. However, they can also backfire and create more problems in the medium and longer term. Eventually, they become part of the problem.

The impact on you of unhelpful behaviours

KEY POINT

Both *helpful* and *unhelpful* behaviours make you feel better in the short term. But the key difference between them is that in the longer term **unhelpful behaviours backfire**. They worsen how you or others feel. So they become part of your problem. The good news is that if this applies to you, you can make changes.

Think about any behaviours you do that are unhelpful.

 What effect do they have on you and those around you, in the short term and longer term?

Choose just one recent example and write down its effect.

Effect on me

Consider the impact on each of five key areas of your life:

Altered thinking: Did it give you a positive view of the situation, of you or others? Were you living according to your values/ideals?

Altered feelings/emotions: Did it make you feel happy/content, or ashamed, guilty, low, anxious or irritable?

Altered physical symptoms/bodily sensations: Was the behaviour good for your body? Or did it make you feel unwell, or put you at risk of longer-term problems like weight gain, an infection, bodily damage or harm?

Overcoming Anxiety, Stress and Panic © Dr Chris Williams 2015

Altered behaviour: Did it help you develop any helpful habits of responding, or keep you stuck in unhelpful or addictive habits of responding?

What other negative impacts are there on your life, in terms of time spent doing the behaviour/activity, money spent, and in terms of what you could be doing differently if you were not caught up in repeatedly acting in this way.

Effect on others

Unhelpful behaviours are often bad both for you and also others.

So, what is the impact on others around you? Was your behaviour good for them? Was it a good example to those you care about? Were they upset or shocked in any way? Will your behaviour stoke up difficulties with others in future?

Some things that may seem helpful but can backfire if you do them too much

Drinking

Having a small glass of alcohol might be quite normal when you are socializing. But drinking too much every day can backfire for:

● *You*: you can get headaches, feel ill, put on weight, make unwise decisions, or your depression can worsen.

● *Babies*: if you have too much alcohol when you are pregnant it can damage your growing baby. Alcohol also gets into breast milk so can harm the baby after birth. Besides this, mothers who drink too much could end up neglecting their baby or harming them.

● *Others around you*: for example your partner, friend or family member: if alcohol becomes a problem, these are the people on the receiving end who will have to pick up the pieces.

The *Alcohol, drugs and you* workbook can help if alcohol or drugs are an issue for you.

Seeking reassurance

Sharing problems and talking things through with people you trust can really help. But if you look to others for support all the time, and contact them again and again for every little thing you do, they may get frustrated. This can also end up undermining your confidence. So what you need is a balanced, supportive relationship.

Seeking (or receiving) too much help from others

Sometimes people may offer 'helpful advice' all the time and want to do **everything** for you. There can be many reasons for this such as being concerned about and trying therefore to help you. Or sometimes it may be because the other person feels anxious or even guilty about your low mood. In a similar way, sometimes people can become almost addicted to seeking approval, praise or advice from others. Constantly seeking reassurance like this is more likely to backfire and undermine your confidence even further.

Whatever the cause, you may feel suffocated and frustrated. Or you may feel that you are being treated like a child. This can again sap your confidence, or annoy you and lead to arguments. And little irritations can quickly build up. The workbook *Information for family and friends – how can you offer the best support?* has some helpful suggestions for you and any of your family and friends to help deal with such issues.

But there's good news. Discovering that unhelpful behaviours are part of what's keeping you feeling low, means that you have now identified something you can change. By working through the seven steps described below you can learn an approach that will help you change any unhelpful behaviour.

Overcoming Anxiety, Stress and Panic © Dr Chris Williams 2015

Have a clear plan

You will need to decide:

- **Short-term** targets – changes you can make today, tomorrow and next week.

- **Medium-term** targets – changes over the next few weeks.

- **Long-term** targets – where you want to be in six months or a year.

That way you can tackle even very big or complicated difficulties step by step.

Overcoming your own unhelpful behaviour

Step 1: Identify and clearly define what you will work on

The first thing to do is to choose just one unhelpful behaviour to work on first.

Look at the following list and tick any activity that you did in the past few weeks. Many different unhelpful activities have been included in the list to help you to think about the unhelpful things that could be happening in your life. You can write in any more you did at the end of the table.

Checklist: Identifying your unhelpful behaviour

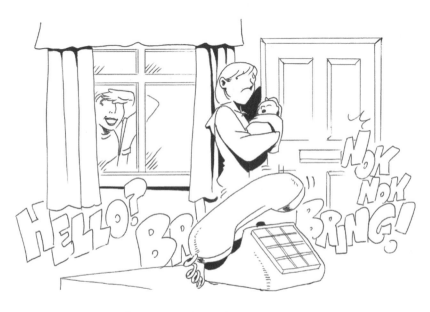

As a result of how you feel, do you:	*Tick here if you have noticed this – even if just sometimes*
Eat too much to block how you feel ('comfort eating') or eat so much that this becomes a 'binge'?	☐
Feel anxious and aware all the time about symptoms of ill health? If you have this problem, you should discuss with your doctor whether you have symptoms of health anxiety or a physical cause of your symptoms.	☐
Make impulsive decisions about important things? For example, resigning a job without really thinking through the consequences.	☐
Set yourself up to fail?	☐
Try to spend your way out of how you feel by going shopping ('retail therapy')?	☐
Become very demanding or excessively seek reassurance from others?	☐
Check your children's health all the time?	☐
Watch TV programmes such as soaps or browse the Internet, etc. to block how you feel – and act as substitute for other relationships around you?	☐
Look to others to make decisions or sort out problems for you?	☐
Drink too much or use illegal drugs or prescribed medication to block how you feel or improve how you sleep, etc.?	☐
Set yourself up to be rejected by others?	☐
Throw yourself into doing things so that you are too busy to think about emotional or relationship issues?	☐
Not let others help you with things?	☐
Look to others to do everything you would normally do?	☐
Lose your temper? Pushing others away by being verbally or physically rude to them? Getting into fights/trouble?	☐
Deliberately harm yourself to block how you feel?	☐

(Continued)

Act in ways that are against your values/ideals? So you live your life in ways you don't like and make you unhappy/guilty.	☐
Take risks, for example cross the road without looking, or gamble using money you don't have?	☐
Check, clean or feel compelled to do things a set number of times or in exactly the 'correct' order so as to make things 'right'? Or do you spend a lot of time deliberately thinking 'good' thoughts to make things feel 'right' or counting good things you've done? If so, you should see your doctor to discuss whether you may have a condition called obsessive-compulsive disorder.	☐
Avoid having sex with your partner because you aren't interested, or because you feel unattractive or angry?	☐

Write down any other unhelpful behaviours you've noticed doing:

Next, use this checklist to choose a target to work on first.

🔍 Example: Paul's target

Paul has low mood and sometimes drinks too much. Everything seems hard, and Paul has noticed he quickly flies off the handle. He has been shouting at his partner Helen. At the time he sees the shouting as letting off steam, but afterward he feels guilty and more down.

Once or twice Paul has felt like hitting Helen but instead he has just left the room. Helen is increasingly worried about Paul, but his temper outbursts are beginning to make her feel angry – at what she sees as unfair criticism. She also feels a little scared. They are drifting apart as a couple as a result, and Paul is spending less time in the house and more in the local pub.

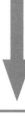

Paul completes the checklist and from it selects one area to work on first.

Example: Paul's target

Paul decides he wants to work on his problem with losing his temper.

Now it's your turn

Look back at your responses and choose **one** problem that you will tackle first. This is particularly important if you have ticked many boxes in the list. It isn't possible to overcome all these problems at once, so you need to decide which **one** area to focus on.

KEY POINT

Often the key is to plan to reduce an unhelpful behaviour. As you do this, consider what will fill the gap. Can you start to build in more helpful responses? See the workbook *Helpful things you can do* for ideas.

My target: Write down a single unhelpful behaviour that you want to change here:

KEY POINT

Remember that this should be a practical or relationship problem.

Break it into smaller steps if you need to.

Be a detective

The next thing is to do some research on your behaviour. First, record your unhelpful behaviour over several days. Make a written note of:

● When it occurs.

● How much and how often you do it (for example, how much you drink, how many times you've sought reassurance, etc.).

● How long it lasts.

Use the **diary** at the end of this workbook to help you understand more about your behaviour. Try to work out what it may be that causes you to respond in this way. For example:

● The time of day.

● Who you are with and how they act.

Overcoming Anxiety, Stress and Panic © Dr Chris Williams 2015

- How you feel emotionally.

- What went through your mind.

- Whether you have slept well the night before.

- How you felt emotionally and physically at the time.

- Any other things you tend to do to cope or escape.

- And anything else that seems to help explain your reaction.

The **purpose** of doing this is to discover more about the issue, and what drives it.

Breaking it down into smaller steps

The important thing is to use a **step-by-step** approach where no single step seems too large. And the first step needs to be something that gets you moving in the right direction. For many problems, you may need to break down your target into many smaller steps that you can tackle one at a time.

 Example: Paul breaks his target into smaller steps

Paul keeps a record of when he gets angry and loses his temper. He realizes that several things affect this. It's often when:

- He has slept poorly.
- When his partner Helen wants to tell him in detail about her day.
- When he has been to the pub.

Paul realizes there are three separate things here he could work on – to sleep better, change how he relates to Helen, and tackle how much he drinks at the pub. He decides to first of all find out more about drink by reading the *Alcohol, drugs and you* workbook. He uses this to help him cut down how much he drinks when he goes to the pub. He finds that the very simple trick of changing every other drink to a low alcohol beer really helps.

He then moves on to working through the *Overcoming sleep problems* workbook. He finds this really helps – and is far less irritable when he has slept better. Cutting the drink also helped that. Finally, Paul returns to this workbook and decides to focus on **how he reacts when Helen wants to tell him in detail about her day**. He realizes he is responding badly to her when he gets home. She is wanting to talk and share her life with him, yet he is pushing her away. He decides to use the current workbook to tackle that.

Now decide whether you need to break your target into smaller steps.

 Is it a big and difficult task? Do you need to break it down into smaller, more achievable steps that you can tackle over the next week or two?

Yes ☐ No ☐

If you answered 'No', then please go straight to Step 2. If you answered 'Yes', then what smaller steps could help you move forward? If you need to, write down your revised first target here again:

 KEY POINT
Sometimes you need to make sure that your first target really is a small, focused problem so that you can tackle it in one step.

Step 2: Think up as many solutions as possible to achieve your first target

When you feel overwhelmed by practical problems, often it's hard to see a way out. It can seem hard to even start tackling the problem.

One way around this is to step back from the problem and see if any other solutions are possible. This approach is called **brainstorming**. The more solutions that you can think of, the more likely it is that a good one will emerge. The purpose of brainstorming is to try to come up with **as many ideas as possible**. And then it will be easier for you to identify a good solution.

 KEY POINT
You can even include ridiculous ideas at first as you are just trying to get yourself to start thinking more flexibly!

 Example: Paul's ideas

Paul wants to work on how he reacts when his partner Helen wants to tell him in detail about her day.
Paul's list of ideas is:

- I could pay someone else to listen to her.
- I could go to another room when I start to feel angry.
- I could suggest we plan a regular time to talk about each other's day.

Example: Paul's ideas *(Continued)*

- We could go for a walk each day and chat as we walk.
- We could plan a half day each week when we could catch up.
- I could ask Helen to write me a letter of what she's done each day for me to catch up in my own time.

To help you come up with a list of possible solutions, think:

Q What advice would you give a friend who was trying to make the same changes? Sometimes it's easier to think of solutions for others than for ourselves.

Q What *ridiculous* solutions can you include as well as more sensible ones?

Q What helpful ideas would others (e.g. family, friends or colleagues) suggest?

Q What have you tried in the past that was helpful before?

 KEY POINT
If you feel stuck, sometimes doing this task with someone you trust can be helpful.

Step 3: Look at the pros and cons of each possible solution

Example: Paul writes a list of the pros and cons of his solutions

Idea	Pros	Cons
1. I could pay someone else to listen to her.	It would be no effort for me.	I can't afford it. It would really annoy Helen. It would also say to her I'm not interested. I really want our relationship to work. I actually want to hear about her.
2. I could go to another room when I start to feel angry.	It would mean I could avoid upsetting Helen by losing it.	She might follow me – we'd end up in a big bust-up.

(Continued)

Example: Paul writes a list of the pros and cons of his solutions (*Continued*)

Idea	Pros	Cons
3. I could suggest we plan a regular time to talk about each other's day.	It would be great if we had a time like that. She would feel happier and we'd actually spend some time chatting rather than having a go at each other.	It would require some effort. I feel so down I'm not sure how long I could listen for. I might get criticized if I forgot anything she said.
4. We could go for a walk each day and chat as we walk.	I know getting out and chatting can really give me a boost. Sometimes doing something can really help me start talking as well.	It's winter at the moment and it's been cold and rainy.
5. We could plan a half day each week when we could catch up.	That could allow us to get the catch up over in a one-off hit – that might be efficient.	Having a relationship isn't supposed to be about being efficient. If things are going to work out we need to start being interested in what we're doing each day – not just have a big tick that we've talked once a week.
6. I could ask Helen to write me a letter of what she's done each day for me to catch up in my own time.	She could write down everything she wants to have me know.	It's a stupid idea. Why would she do that? We're supposed to be partners, not pen friends.

Write your list of ideas into the following blank table, along with the pros and cons of each suggestion.

My suggestions from Step 2	Pros (advantages)	Cons (disadvantages)

Step 4: Now choose one of the solutions

From your list in Step 3, pick an activity that is realistic and likely to help. In making your decision, bear in mind that the best way of making changes is to plan **steady, slow changes**. Choose something that gets you moving in the right direction. Sometimes it's helpful to think of this as one of many small steps that will help you move forward.

KEY POINT

The solution you are looking for is something that gets you moving in the right direction. This should be small enough to be possible, but big enough to move you forward.

Look at your own responses in Step 3 and then choose what you will do.

Example: Paul's choice

Based on Step 3, Paul decides to suggest he and Helen plan a regular time to talk about each other's day.

My choice

Write down your preferred option here:

Check your choice

Now see if you can answer 'Yes' to the questions below.

Is my planned solution one that:

 Will be useful for helping me move forward?   Yes ☐   No ☐

Is clear, so that I will know when I have done it?   Yes ☐   No ☐

Is something that I value, or need to do?   Yes ☐   No ☐

Is realistic, practical and achievable?   Yes ☐   No ☐

If you answered 'Yes' to all four questions, your chosen step is a good choice to start with.

If you answered 'No', then think again and choose another option from your list.

Step 5: Plan the steps needed to carry out your chosen solution

You need to have a clear plan that lays out exactly **what** you are going to do and **when** you are going to do it. *Write down* the steps needed to carry out your plan. Use the *Planner sheet* at the end of this workbook to help you do this.

This will help you to think what to do and also to predict possible problems that might arise. Remember that an important part of the planning process is to predict what would block the plan. That way you can think about how you will respond if there were problems to keep your plan on track.

Now, write down your plan.

 Example: Paul's plan

What are you going to do? I need to talk with Helen about how I'm feeling. I want to say:

- That I don't like having all these arguments.
- That I've been working on that by trying to have less to drink and trying to get some better sleep and that that has really helped.
- That I've noticed that one thing I still find difficult is some longer conversations. I need to tell her that when we chat if I look like I'm drifting off it's because of the depression – not because I'm not interested in her. I'm finding it difficult to keep focused on anything much – papers, TV – anything. So I'm going to suggest to her that I really want to hear from her about what's happening in her life, but can we plan some regular times when we can both sit down together and not feel pressured? Also can we plan to just chat for say five to 10 minutes and not longer?
- And finally that I'd really appreciate it if we could agree that if either of us is just too tired that we can put off the chat for some time later and just be with each other – maybe watching TV or something that feels easy.

When are you going to do it? I need to pick a time to prepare – that's just now – and also a time when we can chat when neither of us are busy. I tend to feel better and more confident toward the end of the day, so why don't I plan to discuss this after tea tonight when we've done the dishes and have sat down for a bit. I'll say there's something important (and good) we need to talk about so she doesn't get scared I'm about to say something terrible.

Overcoming Anxiety, Stress and Panic © Dr Chris Williams 2015

> ### Example: Paul's plan (*Continued*)
>
> *What problems or difficulties could arise?* Just thinking what might block things – there's quite a lot to say and I might forget some of it.
> *How could you overcome them?* I'll keep these notes with me – and practice saying it beforehand. I'll just have to apologize if I look at the notes but I'll explain it's because I want to get things right. Another thing that could cause problems is if either of us feels really tired or ratty. If so I'll put it off for a day and do it the next evening.

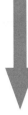

Q What are you going to do?

Q When are you going to do it?

Q What problems or difficulties could arise?

Q How could you overcome them?

Choose a back-up plan

It's good to have a back-up solution for if major difficulties arise with your first choice plan.

 Example: Paul's back-up plan

> Paul decides that if his first choice plan doesn't work, he will plan to go into another room when he starts to feel angry. Because he has guessed she might follow him and they'd end up arguing, he also decides he'll tell her he doesn't want to get annoyed, and that sometimes he will need to leave a conversation for a time, but he is doing that because he is trying to improve how he reacts.

Write your own back-up plan here:

Step 6: Carry out the plan

Your task is to carry out this plan during the next week. Here's where you find out if all that planning has helped you get a good plan. Pay attention to any thoughts and fears about what will happen before, during and after you have completed your plan. Write any thoughts/fears you noticed here:

Try to do your plan anyway.

Good luck!

Step 7: Review the outcome

Whatever happened, now is the time to review the plan and learn from your experience.

Example: Paul's review of his plan

Paul prepares and practices what he wants to say. After tea that evening he brings through a cup of tea for Helen and switches off the TV. He is able to say all the things he wants to (with a little help from his notes). Helen listens and then says how relieved she is to have this conversation. She says that she has been really worried about Paul. She says she hasn't known what to say to support him. She wants to find out more about depression and how she can help.

They agree they will give each other the option to talk less or put off chats if they feel tired or down. They decide they won't see this as a personal rejection – but just something caused by tiredness and feeling low. At the end of the conversation they both feel a lot better. Over the next few weeks, their 'talk-times' help them both feel listened to and supported.

Review what happened with the *Review sheet* (copies are at the end of this workbook). You can answer the same questions below.

 What did you plan to do?

What happened? Did you attempt the task?   Yes ☐   No ☐

If yes:

● What went well?

● What didn't go so well?

● What have you learned about from what happened?

● How are you going to apply what you've learned?

If not:

What stopped you?

- *Internal factors* (e.g. forgot, not enough time, put it off, concerns I couldn't do it, I couldn't see the point of it etc.)

- *External factors* (events that happened, work/home issues, etc.)

- How could you have planned to tackle these blocks?

Use the *Plan, Do, Review* approach to help you move forward.

If you noticed problems with your plan

Choosing realistic targets for change is important. Think back to where you started – were you too ambitious or unrealistic in choosing the target you did? Sometimes your attempt to solve a problem may be blocked by something unexpected. Perhaps something didn't happen as you planned, or someone reacted in an unexpected way? Try to learn from what happened.

How could you change how you approach the problem to help you make a realistic action plan?

Planning the next steps

After completing the first step you need to plan another change to build on this. You will need to slowly build on what you have done in a step-by-step way.

Did your plan help you to tackle the problem you were working on completely? If not, you may need to plan out other solutions to tackle what is left of your problem.

If you are tackling a big or complex problem, what is the next bit to work on?

So, you now have the choice to:

- Focus on the same problem area and plan to keep working on it one step at a time.

- Choose a new problem area to work on.

Steps should each always be realistic, practical and achievable. Without a step-by-step approach you may find that although you take some steps forward, these can be all in different directions. So you could lose your focus and motivation. Use what you have just learned to build on what you did.

Consider your **short-term, medium-term** and **longer-term** targets. This means, where you want to be in a few weeks' time (short term), in a few months' time (medium term) or in a year's time (long term).

Example: Paul's next steps

Paul's **short-term plan** over the next week or so: I want to keep talking with Helen each evening. She also knows that if I feel bad we can put it off for a day and talk then.

Paul's **medium-term plan** over the next few weeks: Helen said she wanted to find out more about depression. Paul decides to give her a copy of the *Information for families and friends* workbook which goes through how to offer the best support. They agree to read through this together each day and also talk about how they both feel. This really helps because Helen finds out a lot more about how Paul is feeling.

Paul's **longer-term plan** over the next few months: I want to look at learning some more ways of calming down when things build up. Paul decides he is going to learn a relaxation technique using the Anxiety Control Module on **www.livinglifetothefull.com**. He gets the free relaxation download from a friend and listens to it on his MP3 player. Both he and Helen find they like using the recording each morning – and it helps them both relax.

Your own next steps

When making your next plan:

Do:

- Plan to work on **only** one or two key problems over the next week.
- Plan to alter things slowly in a step-by-step way.
- Use the *Planner sheet* to check that each step is always well planned. That way, you know exactly what you are going to do and when you'll do it.

Don't:

- Try to start to alter too many things all at once.
- Choose something that is too hard a target to start with.

- Talk yourself out of trying to sort out the problem by saying '*It won't work*' or '*It's a waste of time*'. Try to test out if this negative thinking is actually true by acting against this. Try the plan out and see what happens. You may be pleasantly surprised.

Write your own short-, medium- and long-term plans here:

- **Short term** – What might you do over the next week or so? This is your next step that you need to plan.

- **Medium term** – What might you aim toward doing over the next few weeks – the next few steps?

- **Longer term** – Where do you want to be in a few months or so?

Remember to plan slow, steady changes. By breaking down problems and tackling them one step at a time any problem can be addressed. Use the *Planner sheet* and *Review sheet* to help you get into a system of *Plan, Do and Review*. Copies of both sheets are found at the end of the workbook, and as with all the worksheets can be downloaded from www.llttf.com.

When you need more help

Remember, you are not alone. If you need more help consider asking:

- People around you, whom you know and trust.

- Your doctor/physician, health visitor or social worker.

- Specialist services and voluntary organizations for help with problems such as addiction, gambling, anger and more. They can be part of your plan.

Summary

In this workbook you have:

- Found out about how some things we do make us feel worse.
- Learned some helpful ways to tackle unhelpful behaviours.
- Made a clear plan to reduce an unhelpful behaviour.

Getting more help

The books *Helpful things you can do* describes some habits and responses you can introduce into your life to replace unhelpful ones. If drink or illegal drugs are issues for you, the *Alcohol, drugs and you* workbook might be helpful.

Before you go

Q What have you learned from this workbook?

Q What do you want to try *next*?

Putting into practice what you have learned

Continue to put into practice what you learn over the next few weeks. Don't try to tackle every problem behaviour all at once. Plan out what to do at a pace that's right for you. Build changes one step at a time. Some problems such as drinking, gambling and others may take lots of time to change direction simply because they are addictive.

KEY POINT

Be prepared for setbacks – and times when you slip back into the problem after a period of improvement. Don't get stuck in self-criticism if that occurs. Instead, pick yourself up and keep planning. Don't put off asking for help if you are stuck.

Plan, Do and Review

Whatever you choose to do, the first step is to make a plan and then try it out. The *Planner sheet* will help you create a clear and realistic plan. The next step is to use the *Review sheet* to consider how things have gone – and whether good or bad to learn from it. Copies of both sheets are found at the end of the workbook, and as with all the worksheets can be downloaded from www.llttf.com.

Other sources of support

 www.llttf.com (www.livinglifetothefull.com; @llttfnews)

This popular resource is designed to support readers of this course. There's also a forum where you can make comments, or ask questions of other people using the same course.

Acknowledgments

The cartoon illustrations were produced by Keith Chan, kchan75@hotmail.com.

The terms LLTTF and Five Areas are registered trademarks of Five Areas Resources Ltd.

Although we hope you find this book helpful, it's not intended to be a direct substitute for consultative advice with a healthcare professional, nor do we give any assurance about its effectiveness in a particular case. Accordingly, neither the publisher nor the author shall be held liable for any loss or damages arising from its use.

My unhelpful behaviour diary

Day and date	Morning	Afternoon	Evening
Monday			
Tuesday			
Wednesday			
Thursday			
Friday			
Saturday			
Sunday			

Remember to record every time that you do the unhelpful behaviour.

7-Step problem-solving worksheet

Step 1: Identify and clearly define what you will work on

Select what you are going to work on (your target). Write it down on a separate sheet of paper.

Is it a large or complex problem? Do you need to break it down into smaller steps? If yes, write down your new target on the sheet of paper.

Step 2: Think up as many solutions as possible to achieve your first target

For this step you will need to **brainstorm** possible solutions. Include ridiculous ideas as well. What would you advise a friend? What advice would others whom you respect suggest? Write down all your solutions as you think of them on your sheet of paper.

Step 3: Look at the pros and cons of each possible solution

Write down a list of the pluses and minuses of each option on your sheet of paper. You can draw a table like the one at the end of the workbook.

Step 4: Now choose one of the solutions

Use your answers in Step 3 to make this choice. Write this down on your paper under the heading *My solution*.

Will checking your solution be:

Q Useful for helping you move forward?   Yes ☐   No ☐

Q Clear, so that you will know when you have done it? Yes ☐   No ☐

Q Something that you value, or need to do?   Yes ☐   No ☐

Q Realistic, practical and achievable?   Yes ☐   No ☐

Step 5: Plan the steps needed to carry out your chosen solution

Now, write your plan out using the *Planner sheet* on at the end of this workbook. Include a back-up plan of what you will do if your solution **doesn't fully work out**.

Step 6: Carry out your plan

Step 7: Review the outcome

Use the *Review sheet* at the end of this workbook. Even if the plan wasn't completely successful, there will be things you will have learned. How can you put what you have learned into practice?

Planner sheet

1. *What am I going to do?*

2. *When am I going to do it?*

Write in the day and time:

3. Is my planned task one that:

Q Will be useful for helping me move forward?   Yes ☐   No ☐

Q Is clear, so that I will know when I have done it?   Yes ☐   No ☐

Q Is something that I value, or need to do?   Yes ☐   No ☐

Q Is realistic, practical and achievable?   Yes ☐   No ☐

4. What problems/difficulties could arise, and how can I overcome this?

What could get in the way? Write your possible blocks in here:

Do you need to rewrite your plan to tackle these possible blocks?

5. Write down your final plan here

What are you going to do?

When are you going to do it? (day and time)

Your back-up plan: Think of another back-up solution you could turn to if for whatever reason there are problems with your plan.

KEY POINT
If you feel worse with symptoms you can still choose to do the planned activity anyway – because it's important.

Overcoming Anxiety, Stress and Panic © Dr Chris Williams 2015

Review sheet

What did you plan to do?

Write it here.

What happened? Did you attempt the task?   Yes ☐   No ☐

If yes:

- What went well?

- What didn't go so well?

- What have you learned about from what happened?

- How are you going to apply what you've learned?

If not:
What stopped you?

- *Internal factors* (e.g. forgot, not enough time, put it off, concerns I couldn't do it, I couldn't see the point of it, etc.)

- *External factors* (events that happened, work/home issues, etc.)

- How could you have planned to tackle these blocks?

Use the *Plan, Do, Review* approach to help you move forward.

Worksheets to help you practice *Unhelpful things you do*

Practice is important to help you master this approach. You can download worksheets of all of the key skills used in this workbook from:

www.llttf.com/worksheets/odlm

My notes

Noticing extreme and unhelpful thinking

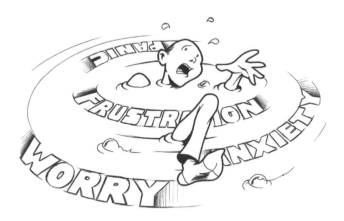

www.llttf.com or www.livinglifetothefull.com 🅣 @llttfnews (public)

www.fiveareas.com 🅣 @fiveareas (practitioners)

🅕 www.llttf.com/facebook

Dr Chris Williams

overcoming
depression and low mood
a five areas approach

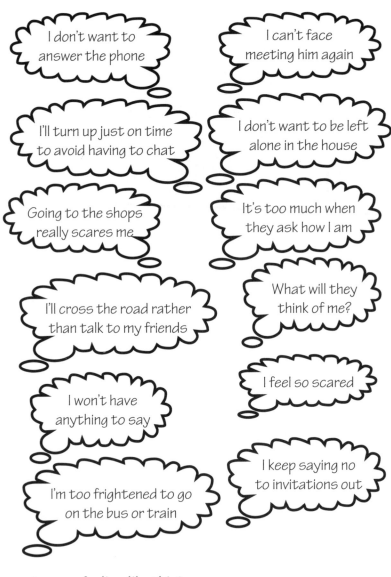

Are you feeling like this?

If so... this workbook is for you.

When you feel low or stressed you can:

- Focus on worrying thoughts and fears – these feelings make you **tense, stressed or panicky**.
- Have unhappy, negative thoughts – these can make you feel **low and sad**.
- Have frustrated angry thoughts about yourself, your situation and about others.

You could also notice **all sorts of upsetting thoughts** about how you feel, your current situation and your future outlook.

In this workbook you will learn:

- How to recognize patterns of extreme and unhelpful thinking that worsen how you feel.
- To watch for habits in your own thinking that are affecting how you feel and what you do.

A second workbook, *Changing extreme and unhelpful thinking*, can be used once you feel you have mastered the content of the current workbook.

Noticing unhelpful thinking

The first step in changing unhelpful thinking is to start noticing how **common** it is in your life.

KEY POINT

Frustration, anger, distress, shame, guilt and feeling down are often linked to unhelpful thinking.

Going through the checklist below will help you to recognize some of the most common unhelpful styles of thinking.

The unhelpful thinking styles checklist

Unhelpful thinking style	Some typical thoughts	Tick if you have noticed this thinking style recently – even if it's just sometimes
Being your own worst critic/ bias against yourself	• I judge myself harshly • I overlook my strengths/ positive things • I dwell on my failures • I downplay my achievements	☐

Putting a negative slant on things (negative mental filter)	• I see life through dark, tinted glasses • The glass is half empty rather than half full • Whatever I've done it's never enough to give me a sense of achievement • I tend to focus on the bad side of every situation	☐
Having a gloomy view of the future (make negative predictions)	• I predict things will stay bad or just get worse • I always expect to fail	☐
Jumping to the very worst conclusion (catastrophizing)	• I tend to predict that the very worst will happen	☐
Having a negative view about how others see you (mind-reading)	• I often think that others don't like me or think badly of me without any reason for it	☐
Unfairly taking responsibility for things	• I feel guilty about things even if they aren't really my fault • I think I'm responsible for everyone and everything	☐
Making extreme statements or rules	• I use the words 'always' and 'never' a lot • If one bad thing happens to me I often say 'just typical' because it seems this *always* happens • I make myself a lot of 'must', 'should', 'ought' or 'got to' rules	☐

Almost everyone has these sorts of thoughts occasionally every day. They become more frequent and harder to challenge when we are distressed. This doesn't mean that:

● You think like this **all** the time.

● You have to notice **all** of the unhelpful thinking styles.

However, unhelpful thinking can affect how you feel. It can also alter what you do.

Where do unhelpful thoughts come from?

While growing up, people learn to relate to others from their parents, teachers and friends. We're also influenced by other things such as TV and magazines. These can often portray a picture of perfection that is impossible for anyone to live up to in the real world. Many people mentally beat themselves up over things they *must/should/ought to* do, or over things they think they haven't done well, and therefore overlook that actually they are doing a far better job than they are giving themselves credit for.

How does unhelpful thinking affect you?

You may believe negative thoughts just because they 'feel' true. This is because of how you're feeling in yourself, and you may forget to check out how true these thoughts really are.

Usually when you notice these kinds of thoughts you may feel a little upset but then quickly move on and carry on with life. But there are times when you're more prone to these thoughts and find them harder to dismiss. For example, when you have some problem you're finding it hard to cope with, or if you're distressed and worn down. At times like this, you may also dwell on such thoughts more than usual. And you may find it harder to move on.

Remember that what you think can have a powerful effect on how you **feel** and what you **do**. Unhelpful thinking can lead to:

1. **Mood changes** – you may become more down, guilty, upset, anxious, ashamed, stressed or angry.

2. **Behaviour changes** – you may stop doing things or avoid doing things that seem too much. Or you end up reacting in ways that backfire, such as pushing others away, drinking too much or using street drugs to cope.

> **KEY POINT**
> Unhelpful thinking styles worsen how you feel.

  Task

The following table shows the links between thoughts, feelings and behaviour. You'll notice in the last column of the table there is a suggestion that *stopping, thinking and reflecting* (**before** getting carried away by the thought and just ending up feeling worse) could help you feel better.

Example: Dealing with unhelpful thinking

Situation	Unhelpful thinking style	Altered feelings	Altered behaviour
You are walking down the road and someone you know walks past and says nothing. They don't smile or meet your eye – they just walk by. Thought: *There's poor Irina – she looks really distracted and upset. I hope she's okay.*	This is normal concern for others. It isn't an unhelpful thinking style.	Concern for Irina	You turn round and catch up with Irina to say hello. Irina looks a little surprised and says she didn't see you. You get chatting and have a really nice talk. Irina has been going through a tough time recently. At the end you both agree to meet for lunch after the shopping to catch up. Stop, think and reflect: *I'm really pleased I spoke to her. She is feeling upset. It was nice to talk – and she seemed pleased too. She suggested we meet up for lunch which is good because it says to me that she wants to see me and enjoyed chatting.*
You are walking down the road and someone you know walks past and says nothing. They don't smile or meet your eye – they just walk by. Thought: *Irina doesn't like me*	This is an unhelpful thinking style: *mind-reading* (that Irina doesn't like you); jumping to the worst conclusion; being your own worst critic; being biased against yourself.	Low/down and upset; anxious in case you meet again	You feel so down you just go home; you avoid Irina in future. Stop, think and reflect: *You never checked out that Irina doesn't like you. Maybe Irina just didn't see you?*
You are at a supermarket checkout trying to pack your bags. You hear someone behind you "tut" as you pack the bags. Thought: *I'm being too slow. They're annoyed with me.*	This is an unhelpful thinking style: *being your own worst critic/bias against yourself*; *mind-reading* that they are irritated by your slowness in packing.	Anxiety; perhaps anger – how dare they – I'm trying my hardest!	If anxious: Maybe speed up packing – fumble and start to drop things. Make all sorts of apologies. If angry: Perhaps slow down the packing, stare at them or pass a sarcastic comment which backfires because you end up in an argument. Stop, think and reflect: *Maybe they were tutting at something else – maybe they'd forgotten to pick up something on their list.*

KEY POINT
Thinking in these extreme ways means that you're only looking at part of the picture. Because of this, these thinking styles are **often not true**.

But what if my unhelpful thoughts are true?

Sometimes we do get things wrong. Sometimes people don't like us. Sometimes we are responsible for a task or someone else like a child. A key is how much we notice these thoughts and how we respond to them.

So, if you have a child, you are responsible for his or her safety and health. But others around you also have a part to play in this. Family and friends may be there to help with encouragement and practical support.

Sometimes when we mind-read we are right – someone doesn't like us, or they judge us poorly. But remember that when you feel low you tend to worry too much about these things – and you worry that almost everyone thinks this way, although there is no reason for this to be true.

Most people are prone to thinking in this way at some time – and even more so when feeling distressed – but thinking like this is upsetting, tiring and affects how you live. The good news is that it's possible to help change things to get back into balance.

Noticing extreme and unhelpful thinking

The first step is to practice **noticing** extreme and unhelpful thinking. You may find there are a number of the unhelpful thinking styles that you fall into again and again. Once you notice these patterns to your thinking you can step back and choose to respond differently.

Here are some examples of how extreme thinking can affect how you feel and what you do.

Example: Sally's unhelpful thinking (1)

Sally is depressed and has tried to avoid meeting people because of low confidence. One day, a work friend phones saying they are all having lunch at the weekend. Sally says she will come with her partner John.

On the day of the luncheon Sally sits at the end of the table and avoids speaking. She mind-reads that *'Everyone else thinks I'm boring'* and this causes her to withdraw into herself.

Sally is also annoyed because John seems to be enjoying himself. She thinks, 'He's more interested in them than me – he doesn't care.' She worries that she doesn't have anything to say and that 'They won't be interested in speaking to me'. She is physically tense – with a rapid heart and speeded up breathing because of her anxiety.

After the main course Sally tells John that she is not feeling well and she would like to go home. She gets up and goes to sit in the car, not saying goodbye to most of the group.

Sally's avoidance and mind-reading prevent her discovering that she would have really enjoyed things if she had started talking to others. Instead she sat alone at the end of the table, cut off from them.

Afterward she is left 'feeling like a fool' for not having talked more to the others – and she is also angry at John. But John is also annoyed with her. He was enjoying the lunch, and thinks that Sally was rude for not saying goodbye. He feels frustrated and criticizes her as a result. They go to sleep that night angry at each other.

Sally's Five Areas thought review of a time when she felt worse

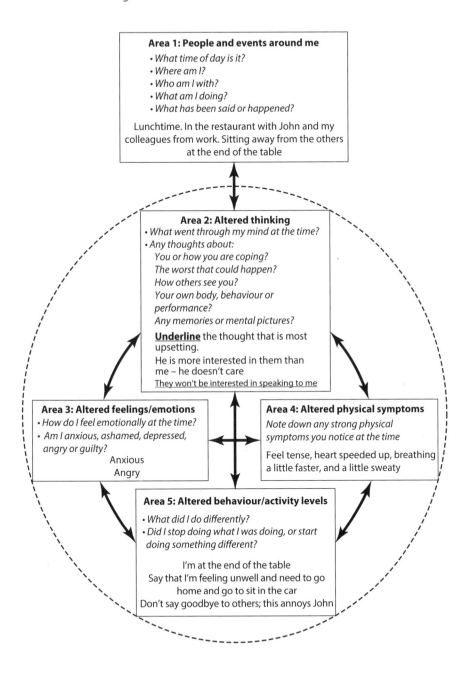

Area 1: People and events around me
- *What time of day is it?*
- *Where am I?*
- *Who am I with?*
- *What am I doing?*
- *What has been said or happened?*

Lunchtime. In the restaurant with John and my colleagues from work. Sitting away from the others at the end of the table

Area 2: Altered thinking
- *What went through my mind at the time?*
- *Any thoughts about:*
  You or how you are coping?
  The worst that could happen?
  How others see you?
  Your own body, behaviour or performance?
  Any memories or mental pictures?

Underline the thought that is most upsetting.
He is more interested in them than me – he doesn't care
<u>They won't be interested in speaking to me</u>

Area 3: Altered feelings/emotions
- *How do I feel emotionally at the time?*
- *Am I anxious, ashamed, depressed, angry or guilty?*

Anxious
Angry

Area 4: Altered physical symptoms
Note down any strong physical symptoms you notice at the time

Feel tense, heart speeded up, breathing a little faster, and a little sweaty

Area 5: Altered behaviour/activity levels
- *What did I do differently?*
- *Did I stop doing what I was doing, or start doing something different?*

I'm at the end of the table
Say that I'm feeling unwell and need to go home and go to sit in the car
Don't say goodbye to others; this annoys John

Completing your own thought review

Now let's look in detail at a particular time when you felt worse. First, try to think yourself back into a situation in the past few days when your mood unhelpfully changed. **Don't choose a time when you have felt very distressed**. Instead, pick an occasion when you were just a bit upset – some tension, or symptoms, anger or guilt. Try to be as slow as you can when you think back through the situation, so that you're as accurate as possible. If you can't think of such a situation, carry on reading. If you can think of one, go straight to the task on that follows.

What to do if you find it's hard to even think about the upsetting situation

Sometimes it can feel distressing going back over a time when you have felt worse. That's why it's important to choose a time that didn't make you feel too upset.

The idea here is to get used to making changes to upsetting thoughts so that you feel less distressed. The key is to practice this approach slowly, with less upsetting thoughts to begin with. That way you can gradually become skilled at jumping in early before upsetting thoughts build up and become too upsetting to easily challenge.

Start to notice the thoughts that link in with feeling somewhat upset. Work with these thoughts first, and use the rest of the workbook to practice changing these. You can slowly work up to more upsetting thoughts later when you are feeling more confident.

 Task

Complete a thought review of a time when you felt worse

Once you have chosen a time when you felt slightly worse, stop, think and reflect as you go through the five different areas that can be affected. Use the blank Five Areas diagram (Figure 12.2) to go through what you noticed in each of the five areas.

1. **Situations, relationships and practical problems**: Think about the people and events around you.

   - Where were you and what time of the day was it?
   - Who else was there and what was said?
   - What happened?

Write the answers in Box 1 of the Five Areas diagram.

2. Altered thinking:

- What went through your mind at the time and how did you see yourself?

- How you were coping (for example, did you think badly of your own self)?

- What did you think was the worst thing that could happen (were you being catastrophic and jumping to the worst conclusion)?

- How did you think others saw you (were you mind-reading)?

- What did you think about your own body and behaviour?

- Were there any painful memories from the past?

- Did you notice any images or pictures in your mind (images are another way of thinking and can have a powerful effect on how you feel)?

Write down any thoughts you notice into Box 2. **Underline** the most upsetting thought. If you like numbers, then you could also rate your belief in the thought **at the time** – between 0% (didn't believe it at all) and 100% (being totally convinced it was true).

3. Altered feelings:

- Were you feeling anxious, ashamed, depressed, angry or guilty at the time?

Write these things in Box 3.

4. Altered physical symptoms:

You may have noticed changes in your body when you are angry or anxious, for example:

- Muscle tension or jitteriness.

- Rapid heartbeat and breathing; feeling hot, sweaty, clammy.

- Poor concentration and feelings of low energy, pressure or even pain. These are caused by the fight-or-flight adrenaline response.

Write these things in Box 4.

5. Altered behaviour:

Was there any:

- *Reduced activity* – you reduced or stopped doing what you had planned to do because it seemed just too hard.

- *Avoidance or escape* – you felt anxious and avoided doing something or left without staying to see if the thing you fear really happened. Avoiding things gives a sense of relief, but often also means we stop doing things.

- *Unhelpful behaviours* – you try to block how you felt by acting in ways that back-fire in the longer term.

Write these things in Box 5.

At the same time, did you also notice that there were other, more helpful, responses that you made?

My Five Areas thought review of a time when I felt worse

Please write in your experience in all five areas.

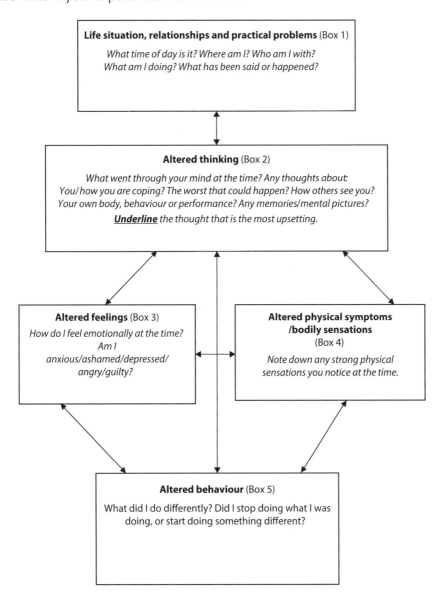

Hopefully, the Five Areas model has shown you that **what you think** about a situation or problem may **affect how you feel** physically and emotionally. It also may alter **what you do** (altered behaviour).

What you think ←——————→ affects how you feel.

What you think ←——————→ affects what you do.

Q Does your thought review show this?   Yes ☐   No ☐

At first, you may find it can be quite hard to notice your unhelpful thinking, but doing the thought review described here will help you to start noticing your thinking. Over time you'll find that this becomes easier. The best way of becoming aware of your thinking is to try to notice the times when your mood unhelpfully alters (for example at times when you feel upset), or when you feel physically worse. When you notice that change ask '*What's going through my mind right now?*'

Remember, we all have all kinds of thoughts during the day. The thoughts we need to change are those that are:

- *Extreme* – that is, they show one of the unhelpful thinking styles described in the *Unhelpful thinking styles checklist* earlier in this workbook.

- *Unhelpful* – that is, they worsen how we feel and/or affect what we do.

Using the thought review worksheet

- Practice using the approach whenever you notice your mood is changing unhelpfully. In this way, you'll find it easier to notice and change your extreme and unhelpful thinking.

- Try to notice and challenge your unhelpful thoughts **as soon as possible** after you notice your mood change.

- If you can't do this immediately, try to think yourself back into the situation so that you are as clear as possible in your answers later on when you do this task.

- With practice, you'll find that you can work out what are the most helpful parts of this workbook for you and use them to help you in everyday life.

Before you go

Q What have I learned from this workbook?

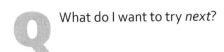 What do I want to try *next*?

Putting into practice what you have learned

It's important you become skilled at spotting your own unhelpful thinking styles. Try to do this several times a day and use the thought review worksheet at the end of this workbook to help you with the task. You can download more from **www.llttf.com**.

Here are some suggested tasks to practice this approach:

- Use the thought review worksheet to carry out a thought investigation on **four** occasions when your mood unhelpfully altered.

- **Stop and think** which unhelpful thinking style(s) you noticed during these times and to **reflect** on the helpfulness and accuracy of the thoughts.

- Begin to ask yourself, *are the thoughts actually **true**?* How could I see things more helpfully and accurately – in a less extreme way?

 KEY POINT
The unhelpful thinking styles are habits of thinking that you are likely to fall into again and again. Just noticing and spotting this pattern can make a big difference to how you feel.

Suggested reading

Once you feel you are able to spot your own unhelpful thinking, then the workbook to read next is *Changing extreme and unhelpful thinking*.

Plan, Do and Review

Now you know what to do, the first step is to make a plan to do it. The *Planner sheet* will help you create a clear and realistic plan. The next step is to use the *Review sheet* to consider how things have gone, and whether good or bad to learn from it. Perhaps use them to plan a time to do a series of thought reviews over the next week so you can get used to spotting these styles of thinking, and noticing how they affect you.

Copies of both sheets are found at the end of the workbook, and as with all the worksheets can be downloaded from www.llttf.com.

Other sources of support

 www.llttf.com

This popular resource is designed to support readers of this course. There's also a forum where you can make comments, or ask questions of other people using the same course.

Acknowledgments

The cartoon illustrations were produced by Keith Chan, kchan75@hotmail.com.

The terms LLTTF and Five Areas are registered trademarks of Five Areas Resources Ltd.

Although we hope you find this book helpful, it's not intended to be a direct substitute for consultative advice with a healthcare professional, nor do we give any assurance about its effectiveness in a particular case. Accordingly, neither the publisher nor the author shall be held liable for any loss or damages arising from its use.

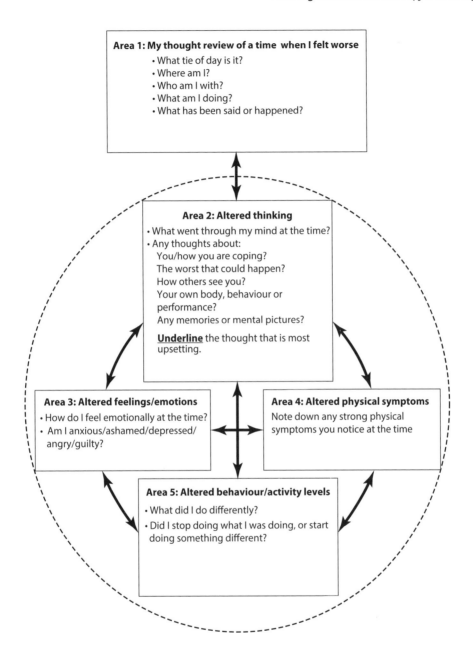

Area 1: My thought review of a time when I felt worse
- What tie of day is it?
- Where am I?
- Who am I with?
- What am I doing?
- What has been said or happened?

Area 2: Altered thinking
- What went through my mind at the time?
- Any thoughts about:
  You/how you are coping?
  The worst that could happen?
  How others see you?
  Your own body, behaviour or
  performance?
  Any memories or mental pictures?

  Underline the thought that is most upsetting.

Area 3: Altered feelings/emotions
- How do I feel emotionally at the time?
- Am I anxious/ashamed/depressed/ angry/guilty?

Area 4: Altered physical symptoms
Note down any strong physical symptoms you notice at the time

Area 5: Altered behaviour/activity levels
- What did I do differently?
- Did I stop doing what I was doing, or start doing something different?

Planner sheet

1. *What* am I going to do?

2. *When* am I going to do it?

Write in the day and time:

3. Is my planned task one that:

Q	Will be useful for helping me move forward?	Yes ☐	No ☐
Q	Is clear, so that I will know when I have done it?	Yes ☐	No ☐
Q	Is something that I value, or need to do?	Yes ☐	No ☐
Q	Is realistic, practical and achievable?	Yes ☐	No ☐

4. What problems/difficulties could arise, and how can I overcome this?

What could get in the way? Write your possible blocks in here:

Do you need to re-write your plan to tackle these possible blocks?

5. Write down your final plan here

What are you going to do?

When are you going to do it? (day and time)

Your back-up plan: Think of another back-up solution you could turn to if for whatever reason there are problems with your plan.

KEY POINT
If you feel worse with symptoms you can still choose to do the planned activity anyway – because it's important.

Review sheet

What did you plan to do?

Write it here.

What happened? Did you attempt the task?   Yes ☐   No ☐

If yes:

● What went well?

● What didn't go so well?

● What have you learned about from what happened?

● How are you going to apply what you've learned?

If not:

● What stopped you?

● *Internal factors* (e.g. forgot, not enough time, put it off, concerns I couldn't do it, I couldn't see the point of it, etc.)

● *External factors* (events that happened, work/home issues, etc.)

● How could you have planned to tackle these blocks?

Use the *Plan, Do, Review* approach to help you move forward.

Worksheets to help you practice *Noticing extreme and unhelpful thinking*

Practice is important to help you master this approach. You can download worksheets of all of the key skills used in this workbook from:
www.llttf.com/worksheets/odlm

My notes

Changing extreme and unhelpful thinking

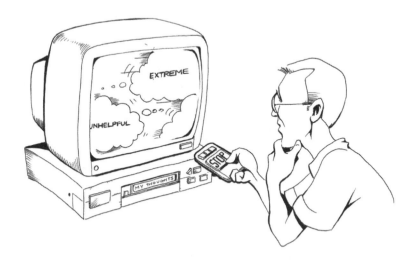

www.llttf.com or www.livinglifetothefull.com 🐦 @llttfnews (public)

www.fiveareas.com 🐦 @fiveareas (practitioners)

www.llttf.com/facebook

Dr Chris Williams

overcoming
depression and low mood
a five areas approach

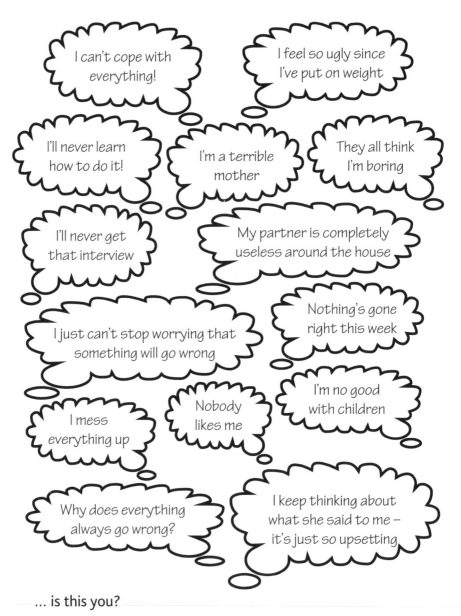

... is this you?

If so... this workbook is for you.

Introduction

This is the second of two workbooks that looks at the area of altered thinking. In this workbook you will:

- Briefly review how your thought review practice went.
- Learn an effective approach to deal with extreme and unhelpful thoughts.
- Use a *Thought Change* worksheet to practice this approach to managing your upsetting thoughts.

Review since the last workbook

In the first workbook in this area, *Noticing extreme and unhelpful thinking*, you were asked to try to do several tasks in preparation for this current workbook. Have you been able to do each of these tasks?

They were to:

- Use the thought review worksheet to carry out a thought review on **four** occasions when your mood unhelpfully altered. Yes ☐ No ☐

- **Stop and think** which unhelpful thinking style(s) you noticed during these times and to **reflect** on the helpfulness and accuracy of the thoughts. Yes ☐ No ☐

- To begin to ask yourself, *are the thoughts actually **true**?* How could I see things more helpfully and accurately – in a less extreme way? Yes ☐ No ☐

Q Have you been able to do each of these tasks? Yes ☐ No ☐

Use the *Review sheet* at the end of this workbook to review how you did.

If you found that you struggled to complete the suggested task, this may have been for a number of reasons. Sometimes negative thoughts may act to block carrying out an activity. This workbook will help you begin to learn new skills in how to alter the negative thoughts that undermine your motivation. Try to use this as an opportunity to change how you think about what you do.

Revision: noticing extreme and unhelpful thoughts

You have already practiced identifying extreme and unhelpful thoughts in the *Noticing extreme and unhelpful thinking* workbook.

You learned to:

1. Watch out for times when your mood unhelpfully alters (for example times when you feel more depressed, upset, worried, guilty, panicky or angry) and then try to notice what is going through your mind at that time.

2. Use the thought review worksheet to carry out a Five Areas assessment of the changes you noticed at the time.

Thoughts that are **extreme and unhelpful** are the target for change in these workbooks. These are the sorts of thoughts that unhelpfully affect how you feel and alter what you do.

How not to respond to upsetting thoughts

Sometimes people try to cope with depression by **trying not to think about it**. Is this an effective strategy? To see how effective it is, try this practical experiment.

Try as hard as you can not to think about a particular object. Please try very hard for the next 30 seconds **not** to think about a white polar bear.

After you have done this, think about what happened. Was it easy to not think about the white polar bear, or did it take a lot of effort?

You may have noticed that trying hard not to think about it actually made it worse and brought thoughts or images of a white polar bear on even more. Alternatively, you may have spent a lot of mental effort trying hard to think about something else such as a black polar bear or something completely different instead.

Conclusion

Trying not to think about something can sometimes cause the thought to become **even more** intrusive and troubling. For many people, trying hard to ignore their worries and not think about them is therefore ineffective and may actually worsen the problem. So there is a need to learn new ways of challenging and tackling extreme and unhelpful thoughts.

Examples of extreme and unhelpful thoughts include:

- "I'm bad."
- "I messed that up."
- "I'll never get better."
- "It's been a terrible week."
- "Just typical – things **always** go wrong."

In depression and anxiety, these sorts of unhelpful thinking styles come to mind more often than at times when we are not distressed. It is likely that when you notice thoughts like these you often tend to accept that they are true. You may notice that it is easier to believe such thoughts at times of highly negative emotion such as when you feel very low, anxious or upset. At times like this, a person is not always completely fair or accurate in the way they judge themselves and interpret what happens to them. It's rare for someone who is depressed or anxious to question the *accuracy* of his or her thoughts. This is important because many upsetting thoughts are extreme and inaccurate as well as unhelpful.

The following skills aim to help you to begin to question the stream of extreme and unhelpful thoughts that may pop into mind throughout the day when you feel low or anxious.

Pick a single extreme and unhelpful thought

To start with you need to pick out a single thought to work on.

- Use the *Thought review sheet*. Choose a thought that is an extreme and unhelpful reaction to something that has happened or that has been said.
- Choose just one thought to question at a time.
- Clearly identify and write down what the thought is.
- For the time being avoid thoughts such as "*I am ..., people are ..., the world is...*" because these sorts of thoughts may be very difficult to challenge at first.

Once you have picked out a thought write it here:

The thought you need to pick is one that is:
Extreme – that is, it shows one of the unhelpful thinking styles.
and is also:
Unhelpful – that is, it worsens how we feel and/or affects what we do.

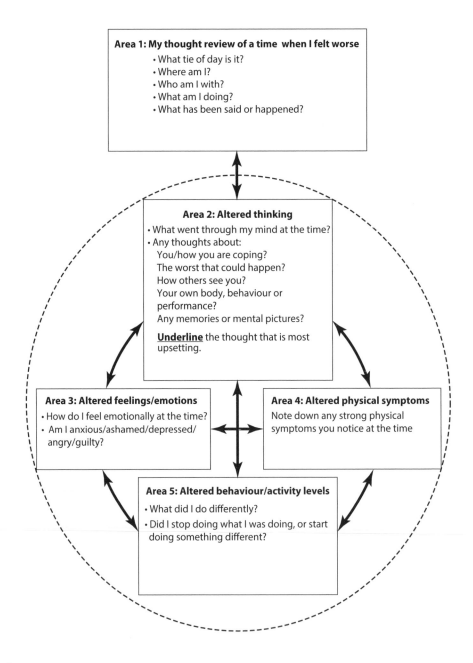

Area 1: My thought review of a time when I felt worse
- What tie of day is it?
- Where am I?
- Who am I with?
- What am I doing?
- What has been said or happened?

Area 2: Altered thinking
- What went through my mind at the time?
- Any thoughts about:
  You/how you are coping?
  The worst that could happen?
  How others see you?
  Your own body, behaviour or performance?
  Any memories or mental pictures?

  Underline the thought that is most upsetting.

Area 3: Altered feelings/emotions
- How do I feel emotionally at the time?
- Am I anxious/ashamed/depressed/angry/guilty?

Area 4: Altered physical symptoms
Note down any strong physical symptoms you notice at the time

Area 5: Altered behaviour/activity levels
- What did I do differently?
- Did I stop doing what I was doing, or start doing something different?

At the time you felt worse:

Rate how much you believed the thought.

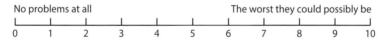

Rate how much it worsened how you felt emotionally.

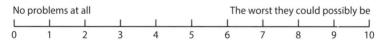

Rate the impact it had on your behaviour/activity level.

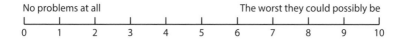

Defusing the impact of the thought

The following five steps are a helpful way of changing the impact of extreme and unhelpful thoughts. You can use as many or as few of the following steps as you need. Just stop when you feel you have defused the impact of the thought.

1. Label the thought as 'just one of those unhelpful thoughts', rather than 'the truth'.

2. Stop, think and reflect – don't get caught up in the unhelpful thought.

3. Experiment. Move on – act against it. Don't be put off from what you were going to do.

4. Respond by giving yourself a truly caring response.

5. Try to act like a scientist: Put the thought under a microscope and ask yourself the seven thought challenge questions (described later).

Let's look at each of the steps one at a time and try out the approach with your own thought.

Step 1: Label the thought as 'just one of those unhelpful thoughts'

Look at the thought you are going to work on. Which unhelpful thinking styles does it show?

Unhelpful thinking style	Some typical thoughts	Tick if the thought shows this thinking style (several boxes may be ticked for some thoughts)
Being your own worst critic/bias against yourself·	• I judge myself harshly • I overlook my strengths/positive things	☐
	• I dwell on my failures • I downplay my achievements	
Putting a negative slant on things (negative mental filter)	• I see life through dark, tinted glasses • The glass is half empty rather than half full • Whatever I do, it's never enough to give me a sense of achievement • I tend to focus on the bad side of every situation	☐
Having a gloomy view of the future (making negative predictions)	• I predict things will stay bad or just get worse • I always expect to fail	☐
Jumping to the worst conclusion (catastrophizing)	• I tend to predict that the worst will happen	☐
Having a negative view about how others see you (mind-reading)	• I often think that others don't like me or think badly of me without me having clear evidence this is true	☐
Unneedingly taking responsibility for things	• I feel guilty about things even if they aren't really my fault • I think I'm responsible for everyone and everything	☐
Making extreme statements or rules	• I use the words 'always' and 'never' a lot • If one bad thing happens to me I often say 'just typical' because it seems this type of thing *always* happens • I make myself a lot of 'must', 'should', 'ought to' or 'have to' rules	☐

> **KEY POINT**
> If the thought *doesn't* show one of the unhelpful thinking styles then you should stop here. Choose another time when you feel more upset, low, angry, anxious, ashamed or guilty and complete Step 1 again until you identify a thought that is an unhelpful thinking style. That sort of thought is a good target for change. Then move on to Step 2.

Step 2: Stop, think and reflect – don't get caught up in it

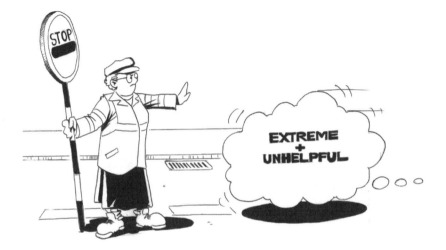

Simply **noticing** that you're having an unhelpful thinking style can be a powerful way of getting rid of it.

- **Label** the upsetting thought as **just another** of those unhelpful or silly thoughts. These thoughts are just a part of what happens when you're upset. The thought will go away and lose its power. It's part of distress – it's not the true picture. You could say to the thought: 'I've found you out – I'm not going to play that game again!'

- Allow the thought to **just be**. Don't allow yourself to get caught up in it. Don't bother trying to challenge the thought or argue yourself out of it. They're not worth your attention. Take a mental step back from the thought as if observing it from a distance. Move your mind on to other more helpful things; for example, recent things you have done well, or even better, on to whatever you are doing at the moment. Really engage in what you are doing so that task is the focus of your attention. Don't be distracted by the unhelpful thought.

Reflect again – how does the thought look now?

Step 3: Experiment – act against the unhelpful thought. Don't be put off from what you were going to do

Unhelpful thinking worsens how you feel and unhelpfully alters what you do. The thought may push you to:

- *Stop, reduce or avoid* doing something you were going to do. This leads to a loss of pleasure and achievement, or possibly to ignoring others. In the longer term it will restrict your life and undermine your confidence.

- Respond unhelpfully, like drinking, to cope. This will worsen how you or others feel.

Make an **active choice** not to allow these backfiring responses to happen again. This often means acting against the thought.

Experiment: If the thought is telling you to avoid something, do the opposite and see what happens. Choose to react helpfully rather than unhelpfully. Choose not to be bullied by the thought into changing what you do. So, if an extreme and unhelpful thought says don't do something – do it. If a thought says you won't enjoy going to that party, go to the party and see if you enjoy it or don't.

To stand up to the bully of unhelpful thoughts, try these dos and don'ts.

Do:

- **Keep doing** what you planned to do anyway. Stay active.

- **Face your fears**. Act against thoughts that tell you that things are too scary and you should avoid them. By taking a step-by-step approach you can overcome these fears.

Don't:

- Get pushed by these thoughts into not doing things.

- Let fear rule your life.

- Block how you feel with drink or street drugs or by seeking unnecessary reassurance.

- Respond in ways that act against your values/ideals of how you want to live.

Example: Sally's experiment

- The next time Sally finds herself mind-reading that others at work find her boring, she decides to not withdraw and go quiet. So at lunch time, instead of sitting in the corner of the room as usual, she sits with her colleagues. She asks them how their weekend went. Everyone is friendly and they have a nice talk. Several people ask what she did on the weekend, and some say that they like her haircut which she'd had on Saturday.
- These actions help Sally change her perspective and feel less anxious. By choosing to go and talk, Sally realizes some important things:
  - First, people were friendly.
- Second, she did quite enjoy it – especially when she was complimented on her hair.

 Write your own experiment in here.

Decide what you will do and when you will do it. Use the *Planner sheet* at the end of this workbook to help you create a good plan.

Step 4: *Respond by giving yourself a truly caring response*

When you feel low, you may often be critical of yourself. People say things to themselves that they would never say to someone they cared for. And they say it in an angry, dismissive and nasty tone. If a friend was troubled by a thought or worry, you would offer words of advice to soothe and encourage them. You would be compassionate to them. How can you give yourself similar compassionate and encouraging words?

Example: Sally's caring thoughts

Sally chooses her Gran. She thinks back to what she would have said. These are words of support and love: 'You know we all love you Sally. People often lose their confidence or do silly things when they feel upset. Don't worry that you didn't chat much with your friends this time – you did well getting out in the first place, it's not worth upsetting yourself about. You can always chat with them later. They'll be pleased to see you – just you see'.

What would someone who loves you say? Imagine you have the best friend in the world – someone who is totally on your side, totally loving and caring.

What words of advice and encouragement would they give you? You might choose a close friend or relative. Or perhaps imagine a famous person from literature or, if you have a religious faith, promises acceptance or support from your scriptures. Whoever you choose, you need feel that the response will be unconditionally positive, caring and supportive. Once you have written it down, also speak it out loud (when you're alone) – and say the words to yourself in a compassionate voice.

Write their caring advice here.

Reflect on this – choose to apply their words in your own situation. Trust what they say. Allow that trust to wash over you and take away the troubling thoughts.

Step 5: Put the thought under a microscope and ask yourself the seven thought challenge questions

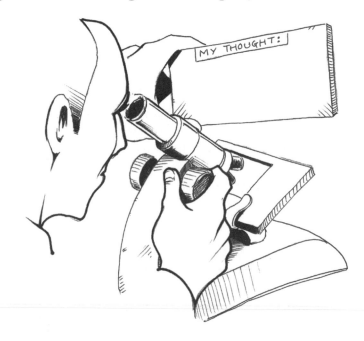

In addition to being extreme, our upsetting thoughts are often incorrect and untrue. Pretend you're a scientist, and look at the thought in a logical way.

Complete the table below to help you work through this process.

Put the thought under the spotlight	Your response
What would you tell a friend who said the same thing?	
Are you basing the thoughts on how you feel rather than on the facts?	
What would other people say if faced with the same thought? Would they be more encouraging to you than you are?	
Are you looking at the whole picture? What might you be overlooking?	
Does it really matter so much based on the wider picture in the world today?	
What would I say about this looking back at it in six months?	
Do I apply one set of standards to myself and another to others? Am I being harder on myself than on others?	

Review the impact of your thought on you now. Look at the thought again. Write it here:

When you think about that thought right now:
Rate how much you believe the thought at the moment.

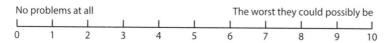

No problems at all · · · · · · · · · · The worst they could possibly be
0 1 2 3 4 5 6 7 8 9 10

Rate how much it worsens how you feel emotionally just now.

No problems at all · · · · · · · · · · The worst they could possibly be
0 1 2 3 4 5 6 7 8 9 10

Rate the impact it has on your behaviour/activity level at the moment.

No problems at all · · · · · · · · · · The worst they could possibly be
0 1 2 3 4 5 6 7 8 9 10

Reflect: Is this different from how you felt at the time? Has your view changed even more during the thought change process? Which of the five steps helped the most? My reflection:

Time to practice

This thought change approach takes practice. You need to practice it again and again until you get the approach into your head and into your life. There are some blank sheets at the end of this workbook to help you with this process. Remember, practicing will really help.

Taking what works for you

When you use the approaches described in this workbook, you'll probably find that some responses work better for you than others. Build on the ones that work for you into your own routine response when you notice upsetting thoughts.

Discussing your thoughts, fears and concerns with others can sometimes help you get a different perspective, and they will no longer seem upsetting.

In this workbook you have learned to:

- Review how your thought review practice went.
- Use an effective approach to deal with extreme and unhelpful thoughts.
- Practice using a Thought Change worksheet to manage your upsetting thoughts.

The approach you have used will work for any unhelpful thoughts that make you feel worse. By labelling, stepping back from and challenging these thoughts, you will begin to change the way you see yourself, the way things are right now and in the future.

Before you go

 What have I learned from this workbook?

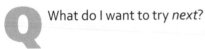 What do I want to try *next*?

Putting into practice what you have learned

There are copies of the thought review and thought change worksheets at the end of this workbook. Make additional copies so you can keep practicing this approach. Pick out the steps that work best for you, and start to use them again and again in your own life. Try to deal with extreme thoughts early, before they become too upsetting.

Plan, Do and Review

The next step is to make a plan and then try it out. The *Planner sheet* will help you create a clear and realistic plan. Then use the *Review sheet* to consider how things have gone, and whether good or bad, learn from it. Copies of both sheets are found at the end of the workbook, and as with all the worksheets can be downloaded from www.llttf.com.

Other sources of support
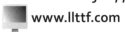 **www.llttf.com**

There are modules here on how to identify and then change extreme and unhelpful thinking, plus downloads of more handouts you can use.

Acknowledgments

The cartoon illustrations were produced by Keith Chan, kchan75@hotmail.com.

The terms LLTTF and Five Areas are registered trademarks of Five Areas Resources Ltd.

Although we hope you find this book helpful, it's not intended to be a direct substitute for consultative advice with a healthcare professional, nor do we give any assurance about its effectiveness in a particular case. Accordingly, neither the publisher nor the author shall be held liable for any loss or damages arising from its use.

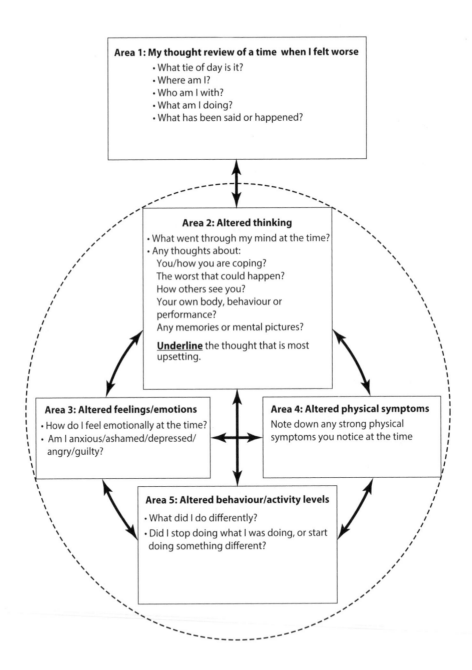

Thought Change practice sheets

To start with you need to pick out a single thought to work on. The thought you need to pick is one that is:

- *Extreme* – that is, it shows one of the unhelpful thinking styles.

- *Unhelpful* – that is, it worsens how we feel and/or affects what we do.

Once you have picked out a thought write it here:

At the time you felt worse:

Rate how much you believed the thought.

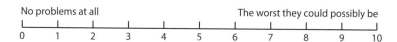

Rate how much it worsened how you felt emotionally.

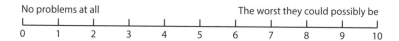

Rate the impact it had on your behaviour/activity level.

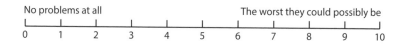

Defusing the impact of the thought

The following five steps are an effective way of changing the impact of extreme and unhelpful thoughts. You can use as many or as few of the following steps as you need. Just stop when you feel you have defused the impact of the thought.

Step 1: Label the thought as 'just one of those unhelpful thoughts'

Look at the thought you are going to work on. Which unhelpful thinking styles does it show?

Unhelpful thinking style	Some typical thoughts	Tick if the thought shows this thinking style (several boxes may be ticked for some thoughts)
Being your own worst critic/bias against yourself	• I judge myself harshly • I overlook my strengths/positive things • I dwell on my failures • I downplay my achievements	☐
Putting a negative slant on things (negative mental filter)	• I see life through dark, tinted glasses • The glass is half empty rather than half full • Whatever I do it's never enough to give me a sense of achievement • I tend to focus on the bad side of every situation	☐
Having a gloomy view of the future (making negative predictions)	• I predict things will stay bad or just get worse • I always expect to fail	☐
Jumping to the worst conclusion (catastrophizing)	• I tend to predict that the worst will happen	☐
Having a negative view about how others see you (mind-reading)	• I often think that others don't like me or think badly of me without any reason	☐
Unfairly taking responsibility for things	• I feel guilty about things even if they aren't really my fault • I think I'm responsible for everyone and everything	☐
Making extreme statements or rules	• I use the words 'always' and 'never' a lot • If one bad thing happens to me I often say 'just typical' because it seems this *always* happens • I make myself a lot of 'must', 'should', 'ought to' or 'have to' rules	☐

KEY POINT

If the thought *doesn't* show one of the unhelpful thinking styles then you should stop here. Choose another time when you feel more upset, low, angry, anxious, ashamed or guilty and complete Step 1 again until you identify a thought that is an unhelpful thinking style. That sort of thought is a good target for change. Then move on to Step 2.

Step 2: Stop, think and reflect – don't get caught up in it

Simply **noticing** that you're having an unhelpful thinking style can be a powerful way of getting rid of it.

- **Label** the upsetting thought as **just another** of those unhelpful or silly thoughts.

- Allow the thought to **just be**. Don't allow yourself to get caught up in it. Don't bother trying to challenge the thought or argue yourself out of it. Don't be distracted by the unhelpful thought.

Reflect again – how does the thought look now?

Step 3: Experiment – act against it. Don't be put off from what you were going to do

Unhelpful thinking worsens how you feel and unhelpfully alters what you do. If the thought is saying to do one thing, do the opposite and see what happens. Choose to react helpfully rather than unhelpfully.

Write your own experiment in here.

Decide what you will do and when you will do it. Use the *Planner sheet* at the end of this workbook to help you create a good plan.

Step 4: Respond by giving yourself a truly caring response

If a friend was troubled by a thought or worry, you would offer words of advice to soothe and encourage them. You would be compassionate to them. How can you give yourself similar compassionate and encouraging words?

What would someone who wholly and totally loved you say? Once you have written it down also speak it out loud (when you're alone) – and say the words to yourself again and again in a compassionate voice.
Write their caring advice here.

Trust what they say.

Step 5: Put the thought under a microscope and ask yourself the seven thought challenge questions

In addition to being extreme, our upsetting thoughts are often incorrect and untrue. Pretend you're a scientist, and look at the thought in a logical way.

Complete the table below to help you work through this process.

Put the thought under the spotlight	Your response
What would you tell a friend who said the same thing?	
Are you basing this on how you feel rather than on the facts?	
What would other people say if faced with the same thought? Would they be more encouraging to you than you are?	
Are you looking at the whole picture? What are you overlooking?	
Does it really matter so much based on the wider picture in the world today?	
What would I say about this looking back at it in six months?	
Do I apply one set of standards to myself and another to others? Are you being harder on yourself than on others?	

Review the impact of your thought on you now. Look at the thought again.
Write it here:

When you think about that thought right now:

Rate how much you believe the thought at the moment.

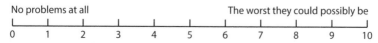

Rate how much it worsens how you feel emotionally just now.

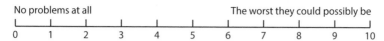

Rate the impact it has on your behaviour/activity level at the moment.

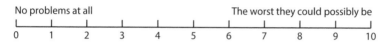

Reflect: Is this different from how you felt at the time? Has your view changed even more during the thought change process? Which of the five steps helped the most? My reflection:

Planner sheet

1. *What* am I going to do?

2. *When* am I going to do it?

Write in the day and time.

3. Is my planned task one that:

Q Will be useful for helping me move forward?   Yes ☐   No ☐

Q Is clear, so that I will know when I have done it?   Yes ☐   No ☐

Q Is something that I value, or need to do?   Yes ☐   No ☐

Q Is realistic, practical and achievable?   Yes ☐   No ☐

4. What problems/difficulties could arise, and how can I overcome this? What could get in the way? Write your possible blocks here.

Do you need to rewrite your plan to tackle these possible blocks?

5. Write down your final plan here.

What are you going to do?

When are you going to do it? (day and time)

Your back-up plan: Think of another back-up solution you could turn to if for some reason there are problems with your plan.

KEY POINT

If you feel worse with symptoms you can still choose to do the planned activity anyway – because it's important.

         Overcoming Anxiety, Stress and Panic © Dr Chris Williams 2015

Review sheet

What did you plan to do?
Write it here.

What happened? Did you attempt the task?　　Yes ☐　　　　No ☐

If yes:

● What went well?

● What didn't go so well?

● What have you learned about from what happened?

● How are you going to apply what you've learned?

If not:

What stopped you?

● *Internal factors* (e.g. forgot, not enough time, put it off, concerns I couldn't do it, I couldn't see the point of it, etc.)

● *External factors* (events that happened, work/home issues, etc.)

● How could you have planned to tackle these blocks?

Use the *Plan, Do, Review* approach to help you move forward.

Worksheets to help you practice *Changing extreme and unhelpful thinking*

Practice is important to help you master this approach. You can download worksheets of all of the key skills used in this workbook from:
www.llttf.com/worksheets/odlm

My notes

Overcoming sleep problems

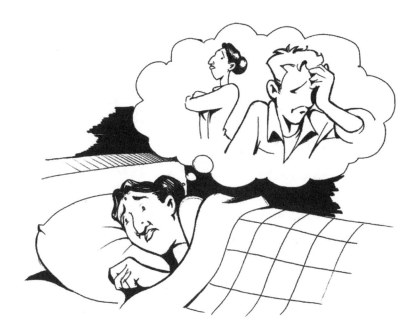

www.llttf.com or www.livinglifetothefull.com @llttfnews (public)

www.fiveareas.com @fiveareas (practitioners)

www.llttf.com/facebook

Dr Chris Williams

overcoming
depression and low mood
a five areas approach

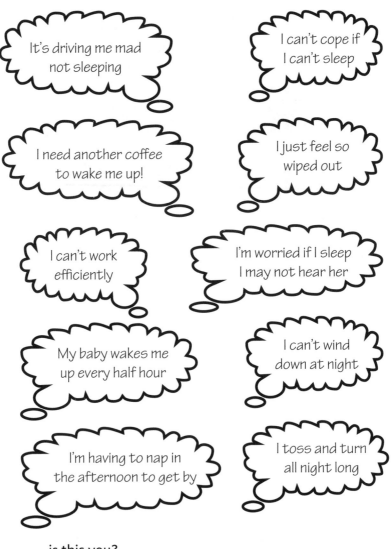

... is this you?

If so... this workbook is for you.

In this workbook you will:

- Learn about sleep and sleeplessness.
- Learn about some common causes of sleep problems.
- Learn how to record your sleep pattern and identify things that worsen your sleep.
- Discover changes that will help you sleep better.

What is enough sleep?

How much sleep you need depends on the person. Some people function well after sleeping only four to six hours a night, whereas others may need as many as 10 or 12 hours. Both extremes are quite normal. The amount we sleep changes over our lifetime; babies sleep much of the day, and older adults need less sleep than earlier in adult life.

What causes sleeplessness?

Most people have problems sleeping from time to time. Sleep problems often start after an upsetting life event, or they can be a result of one's lifestyle. Psychological problems such as anxiety, depression, anger, guilt, shame and stress can also upset sleep. Physical problems such as pain and breathlessness can also stop you sleeping.

A Five Areas assessment of sleeplessness

This section helps you see how poor sleep can affect each of the five areas of your life.

Area 1: Situations, relationships and practical problems

A. Problems caused by the people and events around us

One of the most common causes of sleeplessness is our reaction to things going on around us. External pressures like problems in relationships, arguments, exams, interviews, court cases, debt and more can become a focus.

Q Am I unable to sleep because of things going on with people and events in my life?

Yes ☐   No ☐   Sometimes ☐

If you answered 'Yes' or 'Sometimes', these could be targets for change when you complete the *Planner sheet* later.

KEY POINT

A key decision is whether to approach the difficulty as a practical problem to be addressed, a relationship to be rebalanced, or is to do with changing altered thinking (see Area 2 below).

B. Problems with your bed and bedroom

Problems with noise

Noises that vary or come out of the blue can wake us. If you have noisy neighbours, could you ask them to turn down their television or music? Have you thought about fitting double glazing or secondary glazing inside windows to reduce noise? This needn't be expensive and many reasonably priced options are available.

Your bed and bedroom

- Is your bed comfortable?

- What about the temperature of the room where you sleep? If the room is either very cold or very hot this might make it hard to go to sleep.

- Is there too much light in the room? If bright lights such as streetlights come through your curtains, this can also prevent you sleeping.

Poor mattress

If your mattress is old, can you turn it over, rotate it or perhaps even change it? You may be able to add extra support, such as a board or old door underneath it.

Too hot/cold

If your bedroom is too hot, try opening a window or using a fan. If it's too cold, think about wrapping up with an extra blanket or duvet or wear more clothes in bed. Or you could think about insulation, draught excluders or double-glazing, turning up the heat or using a hot water bottle or cherrystone microwavable pillow for warmth.

Problems with excessive light

Consider the thickness of your curtains. Have you thought about adding a thicker lining or blackout lining? If this may not be possible, for example because of the cost involved, a black plastic bin bag can work well as a blackout blind. It can be stapled or stuck to the curtain rail or window surround. If you use Velcro, you can put this up at night and take it down during the day.

Q Do I try to sleep in a poor sleep environment?

Yes ☐ No ☐ Sometimes ☐

If you answered 'Yes' or 'Sometimes', these again could be targets for change when you complete the *Planner sheet* later.

If you have a baby

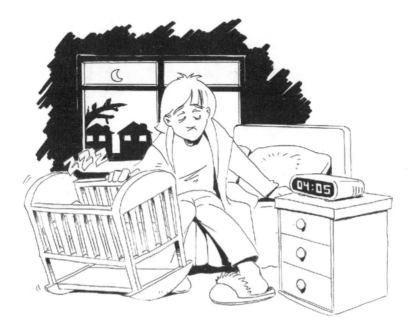

It may take a baby several months or longer to sleep through the night. Also, feeding during the night disrupts your sleep pattern until your baby is old enough to eat or drink enough to see them through the night.

The secrets of the baby whisperer: how to calm, connect and communicate with your baby by Tracy Hogg is a widely recommended book for new parents. You may find helpful advice here in how to establish a regular sleeping pattern for your baby – and help teach your baby ways of settling and soothing him or herself.

If your baby wakes up often during the night and sleeps during the day you should get some sleep when you can while the baby naps during the day. When your baby starts to settle into a more regular sleep-wake cycle you can cut down on your own daytime sleeps.

Area 2: Altered thinking

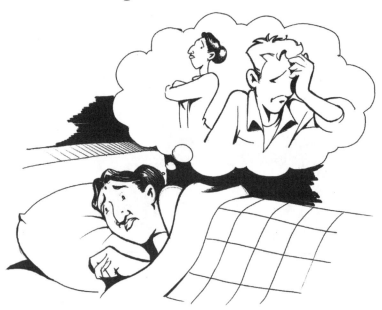

Usually as you start to go to sleep, your tension levels go down so your body and brain begin to relax and drop off to sleep. In contrast, when you're anxious, your brain becomes overly alert. You end up going over things that worry you. This is the exact opposite of what's needed to go to sleep. Worrying thoughts are therefore both a cause and effect of poor sleep.

You may have anxious thoughts about life in general or about not sleeping. For example:

- You may worry that you will not be able to sleep at all.

- You may worry that sleeplessness will reduce your ability to concentrate the next day.

- Your fears then get blown out of proportion and prevent you going off to sleep.

- You may ruminate about things, for example worrying that you may have upset someone.

- You may worry that your brain or your body will be harmed by lack of sleep.

Q Do I worry about things in general?

Yes ☐   No ☐   Sometimes ☐

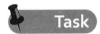
Task

If you answered 'Yes', read the *Noticing and changing extreme and unhelp-ful thinking* workbook. As a first step, write down any worries on a piece of paper by your bed, and mark down a day and time when you will spend time thinking about them. Plan to do your worrying later rather than now while in bed. It's at that time you can then sort out any problems using the *Practical problem solving* workbook.

Q Do I worry about not sleeping?

Yes ☐   No ☐   Sometimes ☐

If you answered 'Yes' or 'Sometimes', write down your worries on a sheet of paper. You can then question any fears that are out of proportion about what the impact of not sleeping will be the next day. When you feel you haven't slept well, see how you feel and how well you function the next day. You may feel tired but your fears that the very worst will happen won't occur.

It's helpful to know that not sleeping enough doesn't have a very big effect on your brain or your body. It is possible to function well with very little sleep each night. When people who have poor sleep are observed in a sleep research laboratory, they may actually be found to sleep far more than they thought they did. Sometimes people who are in a light level of sleep dream that they are awake. So you may be sleeping more than you think.

Q Do I worry about the impact of not sleeping?

Yes ☐   No ☐   Sometimes ☐

Fears about not sleeping can cause increased wakefulness, and actually prevent you going off to sleep. It is important for you to know that these thoughts are extreme and unhelpful. Although you might feel tired and irritable, this doesn't necessarily affect your ability to do things around the house or at work.

Area 3: Altered physical symptoms/bodily sensations

Pain, itching, breathlessness due to breathing or heart problems or other physical symptoms can cause sleeplessness. Tackling these physical symptoms will help with your sleep problems.

Q Are physical symptoms keeping me awake?

Yes ☐   No ☐   Sometimes ☐

If you answered 'Yes' or 'Sometimes', please see your doctor as you may need medi-cal treatment for your symptoms. It may be possible, for example, to change the timing of water tablets/ diuretics that some people take for heart conditions. If you can take these during the day rather than just before going to sleep, this can reduce the times you might have to get up to go to the toilet.

Sometimes if you have depression or anxiety, your physical symptoms can feel worse. Your doctor then may offer you treatment for your low or anxious mood to help reduce the physical symptoms.

Area 4: Altered feelings/emotions

Many feelings can be linked to sleeplessness.

 Do I feel anxious when I try to sleep?

Yes ☐ No ☐ Sometimes ☐

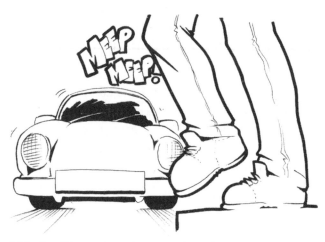

If you answered 'Yes' or 'Sometimes', remember that anxiety is a common cause of sleeplessness. It often triggers your body's fear response causing adrenaline to flow. Adrenaline is a substance produced by your body that makes you feel fidgety or restless. You may notice physical symptoms such as your heartbeat and breathing getting faster, a churning feeling in your stomach or tension throughout your body. Your anxiety therefore acts to keep you alert. This is the opposite of what you want when you're trying to fall asleep. Sometimes you may become anxious about sleeping (for example if you have nightmares or wake up feeling panicky).

 Am I feeling depressed, upset or low in mood and I no longer enjoy things as before?

Yes ☐ No ☐ Sometimes ☐

If you answered 'Yes' or 'Sometimes', remember that depression is a common cause of sleeplessness. For example, when you are feeling depressed you may find that it takes you up to several hours to get to sleep. You may wake up earlier than normal feeling unrested or on edge. Having treatment for your depression can often be helpful for improving your sleep. Other emotions such as shame, guilt and anger can also cause sleeplessness.

Area 5: Altered behaviour: unhelpful behaviours

What about your sleep pattern?

If you aren't sleeping well, you can be tempted to go to bed much earlier or much later than normal.

When people have sleep problems, they are advised to cut down on napping. Napping is a habit that can backfire by upsetting your natural sleep-wake cycle.

A regular sleep pattern can help to maintain a clear start and end to the day. Try therefore to get up before 9 a.m. and to sleep before about 11 p.m.

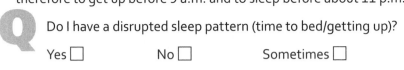

Do I have a disrupted sleep pattern (time to bed/getting up)?

Yes ☐ No ☐ Sometimes ☐

If you answered 'Yes' or 'Sometimes', set yourself regular sleep times. Get up at a set time even if you have slept poorly. Try to teach your body what time to fall asleep and what time to get up. Generally go to sleep between 10 p.m. and midnight. Try to get up at a sensible time between 7 a.m. and 9 a.m. Adjust these times to fit your own circumstances.

Preparing for sleep – wind-down time

The time leading up to sleep is very important. Try to build in time each evening when you relax and wind down. Exercising, eating too much, using the computer or watching TV just before going to bed can keep you awake. Some people watch TV while lying in bed. This may help them wind down, but many people become more alert and it adds to their sleep problems.

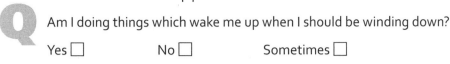

Am I doing things which wake me up when I should be winding down?

Yes ☐ No ☐ Sometimes ☐

If you answered 'Yes' or 'Sometimes', keep your bed as a place for sleep or for sex. Don't *lie* on your bed watching TV, working or worrying. This will only wake you up and prevent you sleeping. You'll also need to decide whether listening to a radio or music helps you go to sleep.

What about caffeine?

Caffeine is a chemical found in cola drinks, coffee, tea, hot chocolate and some herbal drinks. It causes one to be more alert. People can become addicted to caffeine. It also reduces the quality of sleep.

You can get into a vicious circle, in which tiredness causes you to drink more caffeine to keep alert. Then the caffeine affects your sleep and worsens the original tiredness. Try not to drink more than five cups of coffee or the equivalent in one day.

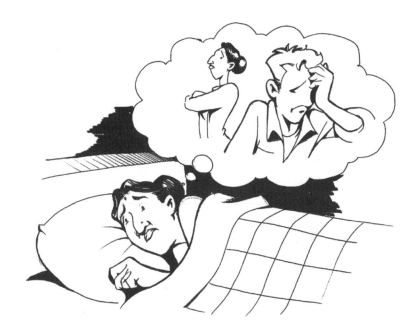

 KEY POINT

Caffeine stays in your body for a few hours before it is broken down by your body or leaves in your urine. This means that you should avoid drinking caffeine drinks leading up to bed.

 Am I taking in too much caffeine or drinking it too late in the day?

Yes ☐   No ☐   Sometimes ☐

If you answered 'Yes' or 'Sometimes', switch slowly to decaffeinated cola, coffee or tea. Definitely don't have caffeine before sleep. Some people find that a warm, milky, bran-based drink can help them fall asleep.

What about alcohol?

Sometimes people drink alcohol to help them get to sleep, but this can actually cause anxiety, depression and sleeplessness. Also, drinking too much alcohol may cause you to go to the toilet more at night.

Am I drinking too much alcohol?

Yes ☐   No ☐   Sometimes ☐

If you answered 'Yes' or 'Sometimes', plan to reduce the amount you drink before going to bed. If you drink above the healthy range, try to cut down in a slow, step-by-step manner. Discuss how best to do this with your GP or healthcare worker.

Unhelpful activities when you can't sleep

Tossing, turning and clock watching

Do you find yourself lying awake in bed tossing and turning, waking your partner up to talk ('Are you awake?...'), or watching the clock?

Yes ☐   No ☐   Sometimes ☐

If you answered 'Yes' or 'Sometimes', then some practical changes can help, such as moving the clock so you can't see it. It can still be in the room so that you can set an alarm or reach it if you have to.

Recording your sleep

You may find it helpful to use a **sleep diary** for a few days. A blank sleep diary is included at the end of this workbook. You can copy out the headings or photocopy the diary and can download more from www.llttf.com. By completing the diary you will be able to identify what important factors affect your sleep.

Carrying out your own Five Areas assessment

Look at the Five Areas assessment in the following figure. Write in all the things you have identified that affect your sleep. These are possible targets for change.

Five Areas assessment of factors affecting your sleep

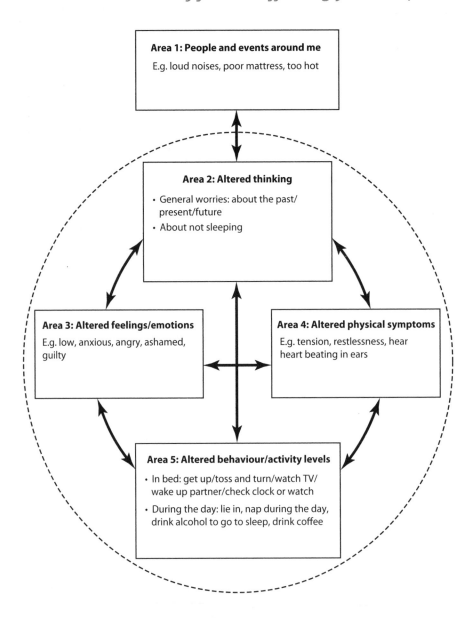

Overcoming sleeplessness

Use the following checklists to find out about things you can do to get rid of your sleep problems.

Sleep checklist: some things to do and not do

Some things to do in the time before bed and during the day	Tick here if this affects your life – even if just sometimes	Some changes you can make and resources you can use
Plan a wind-down time each evening	☐	Warm, bran-based milky drinks may help. Consider a bath/relaxing music.
Have a regular time to go to bed and to get up	☐	
So that you establish a regular body clock, tackle the things that you know affect your sleep environment (for example external noise, mattress)	☐	The *Practical problem solving and Being assertive* workbooks may help you find ways of dealing with these problems. Plan changes to your room/bed as needed.
Reduce your general life pressures	☐	Say no – balance demands you put on yourself. Allow space and time for yourself. The *Being assertive* workbook may help you with this.
Stop, think and reflect on worrying thoughts about the past, the present and the future, and also about sleep	☐	If worrying thoughts keep you awake, write the worries down. Decide to worry or think them through tomorrow during the day. Use the *Noticing and changing extreme and unhelpful thinking* workbook to put your thoughts into perspective the next day.
Live reasonably healthily. People who are fitter generally sleep better	☐	It might sound strange, but overdoing healthy living may become unhealthy, for example doing too much exercise. Try to live healthily but not obsessively so.
Use relaxation tapes or techniques if you find them helpful	☐	You may wish to try the free downloadable relaxation MP3 resources using Anxiety Control Training (originally developed by Dr Philip Snaith) at www.llttf.com

(Continued)

Drinking too much alcohol or caffeine (or smoking) just before bed	☐	Alcohol causes sleep to be shallow and un-refreshing. It can also make you wake up more to use the toilet. Watch out for cola drinks, or too much coffee, tea or hot chocolate, which contain caffeine. Try a slow switch to decaffeinated drinks or water. Don't smoke just before bed; cigarettes cause sleeplessness too.
Doing things that stimulate you mentally or physically in the time before you go to bed (for example using the computer, or watching an exciting film)	☐	You can of course do all these things, but stop doing them at least an hour before going to bed. Avoid doing them in bed.
Let problems build up so that you worry about them at night	☐	Write down your problems to deal with at a planned time tomorrow. Many people find that the worries become a lot smaller in the light of day.
Respond in ways that backfire or make things worse (for example lying in during the day, or napping beyond the time it's helpful)	☐	Try to re-set your body clock by getting up at a set time each day. Try to avoid napping, and to go to bed at roughly the same time each day to get into a regular routine.
Don't look for answers to sleeplessness in sleeping tablets	☐	These tablets are not advisable in the long term.

Don't expect to change everything immediately. But with practice, you can make helpful changes to your sleep pattern. If you find it hard at first, just do what you can.

Your own Five Areas assessment may have helped you identify the problems you have at present. The table above will have provided you with hints and tips in each of your main problem areas.

Summary

In this workbook you have learned about:

- Sleep and sleeplessness.
- Some common causes of sleep problems.
- How to record your sleep pattern and identify things that worsen your sleep.
- Making some changes that will help you sleep better.

Before you go

 What have I learned from this workbook?

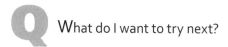 What do I want to try next?

Putting what you have learned into practice

Look back at the **sleep checklist**. From this choose a first target to focus on. Do you want to make changes in how you prepare for sleep, what you do once you are in bed, or change things during the day?

Write down what you're going to do this week, to put into practice what you have learned.

Suggested reading

Various workbooks might be helpful. Think about what affects you the most – thinking, relationships, a lack of assertion, drink, or worrying thinking or perhaps something else. Choose the workbook that you think is most likely to help.

Plan, Do and Review

Whatever you choose to do, the first step is to make a plan and then do (or not do) it. The *Planner sheet* will help you create a clear and realistic plan. The next step is to use the *Review sheet* to consider how things have gone, and whether good or bad to learn from it. Copies of both sheets are found at the end of the workbook, and as with all the worksheets can be downloaded from www.llttf.com.

Other sources of support

www.llttf.com
This popular resource is designed to support readers of this course. There's also a forum where you can make comments or ask questions of other people using the same course.

Acknowledgments

The cartoon illustrations were produced by Keith Chan, kchan75@hotmail.com.

The terms LLTTF and Five Areas are registered trademarks of Five Areas Resources Ltd.

Although we hope you find this book helpful, it's not intended to be a direct substitute for consultative advice with a healthcare professional, nor do we give any assurance about its effectiveness in a particular case. Accordingly, neither the publisher nor the author shall be held liable for any loss or damages arising from its use.

My sleep diary

Time when you are in bed and trying to sleep	Record when you are asleep with a 'X'	When in bed, record any thoughts/images that go through your mind and keep you awake (for example worries, fears about sleeping or the impact of not sleeping)	Record any activities you do that relate to sleep Before bed: alcohol, caffeine, smoking, exercise, daytime napping, computer games, watching scary films, sleeping in In bed: reading, sex, listening to the radio, disturbing other people, tossing/turning, getting up and going downstairs, etc.
8:00 p.m.–9:59 p.m.			
10:00 p.m.–11:59 p.m.			
12:00 a.m.–1:59 a.m.			
2:00 a.m.–3:59 a.m.			
4:00 a.m.–5:59 a.m.			
6:00 a.m.–7:59 a.m.			
8:00 a.m.–9:59 a.m.			
10:00 a.m.–11:59 a.m.			
12:00 p.m.–1:59 p.m.			
2:00 p.m.–3:59 p.m.			
4:00 p.m.–5:59 p.m.			
6:00 p.m.– 7.59 p.m.			

Planner sheet

1. *What* **am I going to do?**

2. *When* **am I going to do it?**

Write in the day and time:

3. Is my planned task one that:

◒ Will be useful for helping me move forward?	Yes ☐	No ☐
◒ Is clear, so that I will know when I have done it?	Yes ☐	No ☐
◒ Is something that I value, or need to do?	Yes ☐	No ☐
◒ Is realistic, practical and achievable?	Yes ☐	No ☐

4. What problems/difficulties could arise, and how can I overcome this?

What could get in the way? Write your possible blocks in here:

Do you need to rewrite your plan to tackle these possible blocks?

5. Write down your final plan here.

What are you going to do?

When are you going to do it? (day and time)

Your back-up plan: Think of another back-up solution you could turn to if for whatever reason there are problems with your plan.

KEY POINT

If you feel worse with symptoms you can still choose to do the planned activity anyway – because it's important.

Review sheet

What did you plan to do?

Write it here.

What happened? Did you attempt the task?   Yes ☐   No ☐

If yes:

● What went well?

● What didn't go so well?

● What have you learned about from what happened?

● How are you going to apply what you've learned?

If not:

What stopped you?

● *Internal factors* (e.g. forgot, not enough time, put it off, concerns I couldn't do it, I couldn't see the point of it, etc.)

● External factors (events that happened, work/home issues, etc.)

● How could you have planned to tackle these blocks?

Use the *Plan, Do, Review* approach to help you move forward.

Worksheets to help you practice *Overcoming sleep problems*

Practice is important to help you master this approach. You can download worksheets of all of the key skills used in this workbook from:
www.llttf.com/worksheets/odlm

My notes

Alcohol, drugs and you

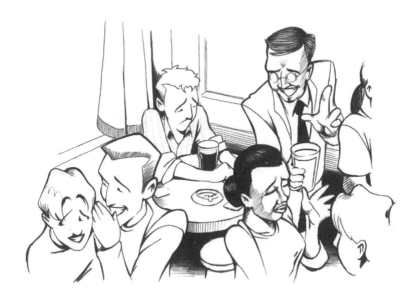

www.llttf.com or www.livinglifetothefull.com 🅱 @llttfnews (public)

www.fiveareas.com 🅱 @fiveareas (practitioners)

🅵 www.llttf.com/facebook

Dr Chris Williams

overcoming
depression and low mood
a five areas approach

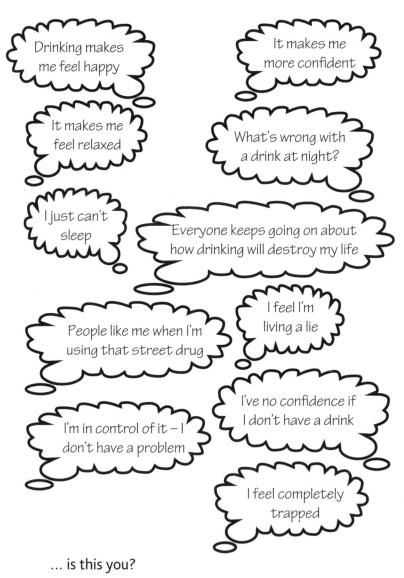

... is this you?

If so... this workbook is for you.

If you are misusing alcohol or street drugs you have a serious problem.

In this workbook you will:

- Learn some useful facts about alcohol and street drugs.
- Discover how alcohol and street drugs can affect you and your family.
- Work out what effect they're having on you.
- Plan some next steps to bring about change if you have a problem.

Alcohol and street drugs are widely used socially – for relaxation and for enjoyment. But they can cause major problems. Also, possessing street drugs is illegal.

Using alcohol

Alcohol is widely used, and is often seen as part of a good night out with friends. However, many people have drinking problems. These often start when people use drink to help them get through.

Have you been drinking to:

- Fit in with the crowd?

- Enjoy the effects of drink?

- Block out uncomfortable feelings?

If you drink a lot of alcohol for weeks or months it can affect your mood, body and relationships. It can also worsen depression and anxiety.

Many doctors recommend that the **highest level of alcohol for adults** to drink in one week should be:

- 14 units for women

- 21 units for men.

The amounts are less (sometimes much less) for younger people, depending on age and weight. Likewise if you have a smaller build, or are older or on medication, the amount you can drink before it becomes harmful will vary.

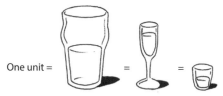

One unit =   =   =

One unit is half a pint of bitter or lager, one small glass of wine, or one measure of spirits (for example, whisky or gin). These values vary because stronger lagers or beers, or fortified wines, contain more than one unit of alcohol.

> **KEY POINT**
>
> Always look at the back of the bottle, where you'll find how many units of alcohol there are in a standard size glass for that particular drink. You can also work it out using the online calculator available at **http://www.nhs.uk /Tools/Pages/Alcoholcalculator.aspx**.

The key is whether you are experiencing *harmful drinking*. If you are, no matter how many units you drink a week, you need to cut back. Doctors now recommend that if you drink, you plan to have at least two drink-free days a week to allow your body to cleanse itself and recover from the impact of drink.

Street drugs

There are many different street drugs and they are usually used for similar reasons to drinking alcohol. Possession of street drugs is illegal because the risks of using them are higher than alcohol and there is no regulation so doses and content can vary dangerously. Even when you think you may be buying one type of drug on the street, it may be contaminated with other drugs or substances. These drugs can have sudden and extreme negative impacts on mental (and physical) health. The effects of different drugs vary, but some effects are common to all drugs and alcohol.

 For more information about street drugs, visit the Talk to Frank website (**www.talktofrank.com**).

Recording the drink and drugs you use

 Task

Whether you are drinking or taking street drugs, a **good first step** is to record how much you use. Most people tend to think they have taken or drank a lot less than they actually have.

 How many units of alcohol do you drink?

In one day:

- What drink? _____

- How much? _____

- How many times? _____

In one week?

- What drink? _____

  - How much? _____

  - How many times? _____

How many units is that per week? _____ units

How much are you spending a week on drinks? _____

What street drugs are you taking?

In one day:

  - What drug? _____

  - How much? _____

  - How many times? _____

In one week?

  - What drug? _____

  - How much? _____

  - How many times? _____

How much are you spending per week on drugs? _____

The best way of finding out how much you drink or use in a week is to keep a **diary**. You'll find one at the back of this workbook. Try to **record every time** you drink alcohol or use drugs. At the end of the week, add up the amount and cost of what you have taken.

How alcohol and drugs affect you

When you drink a large amount of alcohol or take a large dose of drugs – or regularly drink or take drugs at low doses – you can be harmed. Some of these are described below.

Thinking/psychological harm

People often drink or use drugs to improve how they feel. But actually these can cause anxiety and low mood, and prevent your depression getting better.

Drinking and taking drugs can:

● Worsen worry and panic attacks.

● Lead to sudden bouts of confusion or violence.

- Damage your concentration and memory, so that you find it hard to learn and remember new information.

- Impact your ability to fall asleep and to have a refreshing night's sleep.

- Cause you to become fearful, increasingly suspicious and mistrustful of others.

- Lead to addiction, with craving if you stop taking them abruptly.

Drinking and taking drugs can make you feel irritable. Your personality changes, in such a subtle way that you may not realize that you're changing as a result of your habit. You can become withdrawn, stop taking interest in other people or the things around you. You could become suspicious of everything around you.

People can develop severe psychiatric (mental health) disorders that can become long term, such as having hallucinations (seeing or hearing things that aren't there) or delusions (believing something is true when it isn't). These illnesses can be terrifying.

Q Do you have any of the mental health symptoms described above? (**Note**: You may need to ask people around you.)

Yes ☐   No ☐   Sometimes ☐

Physical changes

- The most common symptom of drinking too much is having a hangover. You feel sick, with headaches, and are dehydrated.

- Both alcohol and drugs can lead to addiction. If you suddenly stop either, you may notice **withdrawal symptoms** such as being sweaty and feeling sick. If you take a lot of alcohol or drugs, you can become dependent on them. You can also become dependent on the so-called 'soft' drugs, for example cannabis – some types of which are not 'soft' in effect at all.

- If someone drinks or uses drugs at a high level for some time and then suddenly stops them, there is a high risk of withdrawal. This is a serious medical condition. Symptoms of withdrawal include confusion, agitation and hallucinations. The person can go into a coma, have fits or wet themselves.

- Alcohol causes damage to parts of the body. It can cause stomach ulcers (holes in the lining of the stomach) and liver. It can also damage the brain, leading to epileptic fits. Other important body organs such as the pancreas can be damaged, causing pain.

- Drugs can lead to lung cancer and heart problems, or possible stroke. Epileptic fits are possible, or body temperature regulation can be upset. They can cause confusion and at worst, sudden death.

- Taking drugs can reduce the ability to fight off infections or serious disease.

Overcoming Anxiety, Stress and Panic © Dr Chris Williams 2015

Q Do you have any of the physical symptoms described above?

Yes ☐ No ☐ Sometimes ☐

Social changes

● When drink and drugs take hold they have a powerful impact on how you live your life. You may start to forget your values and ideals of how you want to live, and the drink or drugs become the most important thing in your life. Other important things get pushed out as a result.

● You may have problems at home such as **arguments** with family and friends.

● You may get into **debt**.

● You may struggle to keep up at work – or with the house. You may ignore or neglect people you care about such as your partner, children or friends.

● **Accidents and violence** are also common social consequences of alcohol dependency.

Q Do you have any of the social changes described above?

Yes ☐ No ☐ Sometimes ☐

Based on your answers to all the questions above:

Overall, do you think that you're having drink/drug problems?

Yes ☐ No ☐ Sometimes ☐

If you have answered 'Yes' or 'Sometimes' to this question, this is an alert that you need to make some changes.

> **KEY POINT**
> Drinking or using drugs in ways that can harm you or others is likely to cause increasing problems in each of the areas described above. You need to tackle your problem now. Don't be tempted to downplay or ignore things and pretend there isn't a problem. Ignoring obvious signs is often part of the problem.

Paul has started to drink more to try to cope with symptoms of low mood. His drinking is now affecting both him and his partner Helen. But Paul doesn't think he has a drinking problem. He sees drink as something that is *helpful*. This is because he hasn't worked out the harmful effects of the drinking on his life. He needs to start looking at the **downsides** of his drinking as well as the immediate perceived benefits. This means looking at the short-term and longer-term effects of his daily drinking on himself and on his partner.

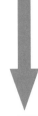

Is your drinking harming you?

Example: Is Paul's drinking harming him?

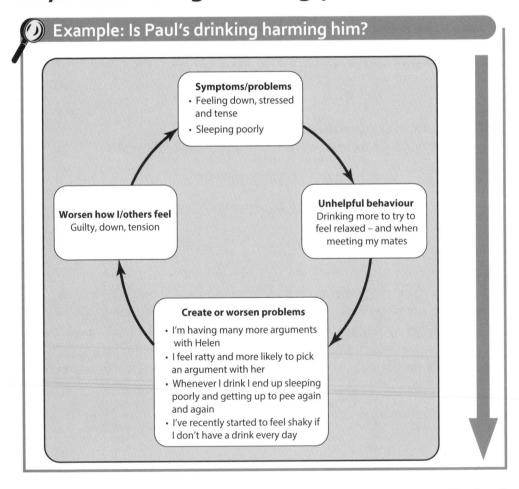

Symptoms/problems
- Feeling down, stressed and tense
- Sleeping poorly

Unhelpful behaviour
Drinking more to try to feel relaxed – and when meeting my mates

Create or worsen problems
- I'm having many more arguments with Helen
- I feel ratty and more likely to pick an argument with her
- Whenever I drink I end up sleeping poorly and getting up to pee again and again
- I've recently started to feel shaky if I don't have a drink every day

Worsen how I/others feel
Guilty, down, tension

(Continued)

Example: Is Paul's drinking harming him? *(Continued)*

In the short term:

- **Physically:** Paul is noticing he *feels shaky* if he doesn't have a drink every day.
- **Psychologically:** He feels drinking makes him more relaxed and helps him fall asleep at night. But then he *wakes up* and has to go to the toilet. So he *feels too tired to get up in the morning* and *sleeps in* to catch up on sleep. This worsens his sleeping pattern. He also feels *more depressed* in the morning when he's been drinking the night before.
- **Socially:** Paul's *partner Helen is worried about him.* They *keep having arguments* about this. Paul knows it's *damaging their relationship.*

 KEY POINT

Both *helpful* and *unhelpful* behaviours may make us feel better in the short term. But in the longer term, our unhelpful behaviours such as heavy drinking backfire. They worsen how we or others feel. They become part of our problem.

The good news is that if this applies to you, you can make changes.

 Task

Now think about your own drinking or drug use or both.

How does my drinking or drug use affect me and the people around me in the short term and longer term?

Short term

- Physically.

- Psychologically.

- Socially (on you and others for example, your family, children, friends).

Longer term (look back to over the past 6 to 12 months)

- Physically.

- Psychologically.

- Socially (on you and others).

If after reading this workbook you have discovered that your drinking or drug use is causing harm to you or others, then **you need to tackle it**.

How to make changes

Try to reduce your overall intake of alcohol or drugs each week.

- Do this slowly in steady steps over several weeks.
- If possible, plan to eventually have **at least two days** each week without any drink or drugs to allow your body to recover.

Discuss your goals and how to achieve this with your doctor.

If you're drinking or using street drugs at a higher level

If you stop drinking or taking the drugs too quickly, you may notice some symptoms of withdrawal. This is probably why so many people don't manage to tackle this problem. But it's possible to make changes – and it's even more important to do so if you're drinking or using drugs at this level.

To change successfully you need to cut down the amount you're taking in a **slow, step-by-step manner**. You may find the *Unhelpful things you do* workbook helpful for some ideas of how to plan this. But if you're taking drugs or drinking alcohol at higher levels, it's best to make these changes together with help and advice from your GP, health visitor, your local drug or alcohol support services or other healthcare practitioner.

KEY POINT

If you regularly use street drugs or drink a lot of alcohol, please can you discuss this with someone who can help.

Summary

In this workbook you have learned:

- Some useful facts about alcohol and street drugs.
- How alcohol and street drugs can affect you and your family.
- How you can work out what effects they're having on you.
- How to plan some next steps to bring about change if you have a problem.

Q What have I learned from this workbook?

Q What do I want to try *next*?

Putting into practice what you have learned

You are likely to make the most progress if you can act on what you have learned in the workbook. It may be tempting to put it off. It may be really hard to change because of the grip that drink has on you. That's when you need extra help. Ask your GP about local support groups such as Alcoholics Anonymous and local Drink and Drug services.

Plan, Do and Review

Whatever you choose to do, the first step is to make a plan and then do (or not do) it. The *Planner sheet* will help you create a clear and realistic plan. The next step is to use the *Review sheet* to consider how things have gone, and whether good or bad to learn from it. Copies of both sheets are found at the end of the workbook, and as with all the worksheets can be downloaded from www.llttf.com.

Other sources of support

Ask your GP, and look at your local directory and also search online for local support services.

Acknowledgments

The cartoon illustrations were produced by Keith Chan, kchan75@hotmail.com.

The terms LLTTF and Five Areas are registered trademarks of Five Areas Resources Ltd.

Although we hope you find this book helpful, it's not intended to be a direct substitute for consultative advice with a healthcare professional, nor do we give any assurance about its effectiveness in a particular case. Accordingly, neither the publisher nor the author shall be held liable for any loss or damages arising from its use.

Drink/street drug diary: my week

Day and date	Morning	Afternoon	Evening	Total units or cost
Monday				Total units/amount per day = Cost/day =
Tuesday				Total units/amount per day = Cost/day =
Wednesday				Total units/amount per day = Cost/day =
Thursday				Total units/amount per day = Cost/day =
Friday				Total units/amount per day = Cost/day =
Saturday				Total units/amount per day = Cost/day =
Sunday				Total units/amount per day = Cost/day =
Weekly total				Units =
Cost =				

Note: Remember to record everything you drink/take. If you are drinking/using drugs on a regular basis and/or at a high dose, it may prevent you getting better.

Planner sheet

1. *What* am I going to do?

2. *When* am I going to do it?

Write in the day and time:

3. Is my planned task one that:

Ｑ Will be useful for helping me move forward?	Yes ☐	No ☐
Ｑ Is clear, so that I will know when I have done it?	Yes ☐	No ☐
Ｑ Is something that I value, or need to do?	Yes ☐	No ☐
Ｑ Is realistic, practical and achievable?	Yes ☐	No ☐

4. What problems/difficulties could arise, and how can I overcome this?

What could get in the way? Write your possible blocks in here.

Do you need to rewrite your plan to tackle these possible blocks?

5. Write down your final plan here.

What are you going to do?

When are you going to do it? (day and time)

Your back-up plan: Think of another back-up solution you could turn to if for whatever reason there are problems with your plan.

KEY POINT
If you feel worse with symptoms you can still choose to do the planned activity anyway – because it's important.

Overcoming Anxiety, Stress and Panic © Dr Chris Williams 2015

Review sheet

What did you plan to do?

Write it here.

What happened? Did you attempt the task?   Yes ☐   No ☐

If yes:

● What went well?

● What didn't go so well?

● What have you learned about from what happened?

● How are you going to apply what you've learned?

If not:

What stopped you?

● *Internal factors* (e.g. forgot, not enough time, put it off, concerns I couldn't do it, I couldn't see the point of it, etc.)

● *External factors* (events that happened, work/home issues, etc.)

● How could you have planned to tackle these blocks?

Use the *Plan, Do, Review* approach to help you move forward.

Worksheets to help you practice *Alcohol, drugs and you*

Practice is important to help you master this approach. You can download worksheets of all of the key skills used in this workbook from:

www.llttf.com/worksheets /odlm

My notes

Understanding and using antidepressant medication

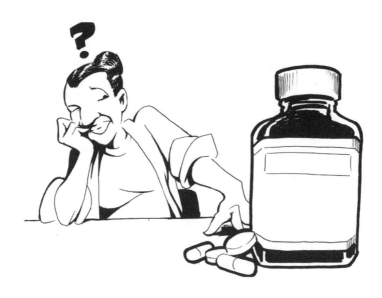

www.llttf.com or www.livinglifetothefull.com 🅑 @llttfnews (public)

www.fiveareas.com 🅑 @fiveareas (practitioners)

f www.llttf.com/facebook

Dr Chris Williams

overcoming
depression and low mood
a five areas approach

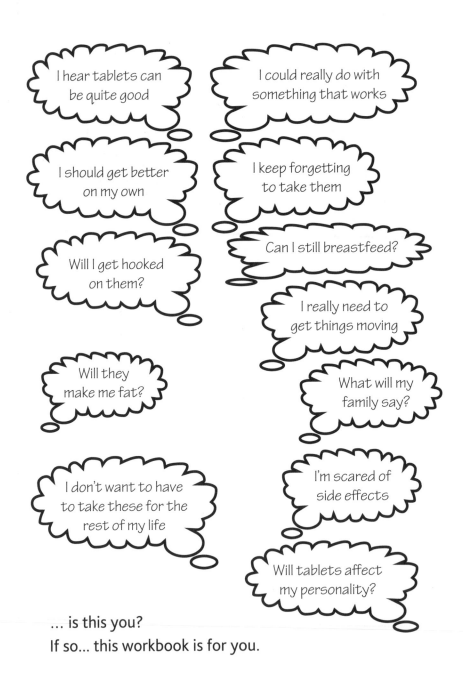

... is this you?

If so... this workbook is for you.

In this workbook you will:

- Find out about how antidepressants are used for clinical depression.
- Get the answers to some common questions about antidepressants.
- Get some useful hints and tips to get the best out of your medication.
- Learn how to think through the pros and cons of medication if it is suggested for you.

How do antidepressant medications fit in with your treatment?

Antidepressant medications can be helpful as part of a **package of care**. National guidelines often recommend that people with depression should be offered treatment such as psychological or 'talking' treatment as well as medication. They can both be equal parts of a package of care. Your doctor can tell you more about the different types of antidepressants available.

KEY POINT

If you're already using an antidepressant you shouldn't stop them if they are helping. Continue to take them as originally planned. All of your treatment decisions should be made with your doctor.

When are antidepressants helpful?

Antidepressants are at their most helpful if you have moderate or severe symptoms of depression. This is sometimes called **clinical depression** – a situation in which your depression is having a major effect on your life. Symptoms of clinical depression include:

- Feeling low or noticing you no longer enjoy things most of the time for at least two weeks.

- Physical changes such as low energy, reduced concentration, changes in your sleep pattern or appetite.

- Feeling very agitated, suspicious or panicky.

- Noticing suicidal ideas, that is, where you have no hope for the future.

When are antidepressants not helpful?

Usually antidepressants aren't meant for problems of mildly low mood, but they may be prescribed for symptoms that persist and are troubling.

Some other times when antidepressants may be used

In addition to clinical depression, antidepressants are sometimes used to treat other mental and physical health problems. For example:

- Anxiety and tension

- Panic attacks

- Physical symptoms such as chronic fatigue (feeling tired all the time), fibromyalgia (pain in muscles and joints) and general body aches

- Obsessive-compulsive disorder (OCD)

KEY POINT
Ask your doctor the reason why you may be prescribed an antidepressant and how long you might need to take them for.

Your attitudes toward medication

I think I should get better on my own without medication

Taking antidepressant medications is one of many important ways of helping you to get better. They can help with some of the physical symptoms that may be part of clinical depression. They boost how you feel. However, taking antidepressants doesn't replace the need for you to work at changing other things in your life, such as relationship problems or other practical problems.

KEY POINT
Remember, our body, thoughts and feelings are all part of us – they are not in separate boxes. If you break your leg, you are unlikely to say 'I want to get better by myself without medical treatment'. So why do this if you're experiencing depression? If your doctor recommends that you take antidepressants, discuss the reasons for suggesting this. You should jointly make the decision about whether it's the right thing for you at the moment.

My family and friends are unhappy I'm taking medication

Sometimes people have strong views about antidepressants. As in the example above about the broken leg, the best advice is that if your doctor suggests a treatment that's known to work well, you should try it. This won't always mean taking medication, although medication can often be an important part of an overall treatment package. If your friends or family continue to be unhappy about this, perhaps you could discuss this with them through the content of this workbook, or ask them to come with you to discuss their concerns with your doctor.

Frequently asked questions

Why do doctors use antidepressant medication for treating depression?

Remember the Five Areas model: in depression there are links between the changes in your thinking, feelings, behaviour and your body. Because of the links between each of the areas, the **physical treatment** offered by medication can lead to improvements in the other areas too.

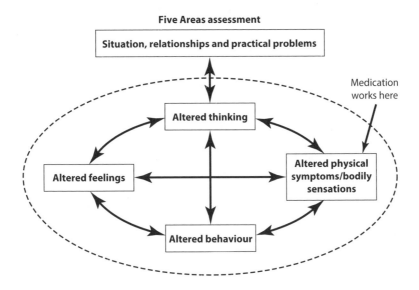

How well do antidepressant tablets work?

About two-thirds of people who have severe or moderate depression find that taking antidepressants helps with their symptoms.

How long do they take to work?

Don't expect immediate results. Antidepressant medicines can take up to two to four weeks to begin to work. And it may take longer for their full effects to show. Therefore it's very important that you take the tablets regularly and for long enough, even if at first it doesn't feel like they doing anything. Sometimes doctors advise a low dose to start with. This can be slowly increased over several weeks/months if needed.

KEY POINT
You shouldn't give up on your antidepressant medicine if you don't notice changes straight away.

  Do antidepressants have side effects?

All medications have side effects. That is true of aspirin and paracetamol as well as antidepressants. The important question is whether the effects of having untreated depression are worse. Most modern antidepressant medicines that are used for clinical depression have fewer side effects than antidepressants that were prescribed 20 to 30 years ago. For example, they usually don't cause significant drowsiness.

Many side effects improve within a few days of starting the tablets as your body gets used to them. Sometimes anxiety can increase how much we notice our symptoms. Your doctor should go through the possible side effects with you when you start treatment, but you can always ask them again if you are unsure. You can also read the patient information leaflet that comes with every prescription.

  Can I drive or use machinery if I take antidepressants?

Many antidepressant medications can affect your ability to drive and operate machinery. They can also increase the effects of alcohol. Read the patient information leaflet that you receive with your prescription to see if this applies, or ask your doctor if you have any doubts.

  Are antidepressants addictive?

Antidepressants are not addictive in the way that some other drugs are, but stopping them suddenly may cause unpleasant symptoms. Because of this, when you are ready to stop taking the tablets your doctor may suggest you taper down the dose over several weeks or months. It's important to take medical advice when reducing and stopping antidepressants.

What if I might be pregnant?

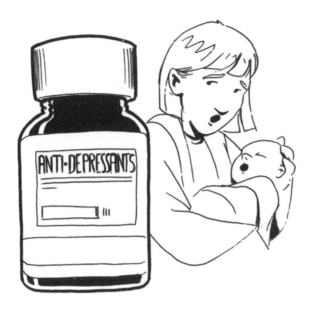

If you're pregnant you may worry about taking medications. If you are already on medication then you need to discuss this with your doctor.

So if you think you may be pregnant, **tell your doctor straight away**. Sometimes your doctor may suggest starting antidepressants during pregnancy. You and your doctor will balance the pros and cons of this for you and your unborn baby. Remember it's also important for your baby that you are getting the most appropriate treatment for your depression and that you stay well to look after your baby when he or she is born.

 Can I breastfeed and also take an antidepressant?

If you are breastfeeding, some of the medication may pass in the milk to your baby. It's usually possible for your doctor to choose an antidepressant that is less likely to be passed along to your baby if you are nursing, or you may choose not to breastfeed if it is more important to stay on the medication.

Practical problems you may have while taking medication

Remembering to take your medication

It can be hard to remember to take any medication on a regular basis. It's even harder when depression affects your concentration. You might want to try these methods.

- Many tablets come in blister packs that state the day or time of day to take the tablets.

- Get into a routine. Take the tablets at a set time each day.

- Many chemists/pharmacies sell plastic pill organizers (sometimes called dosette boxes) that have compartments for each day and part of the day into which you can place the correct doses of tablets. That way you will know when you have taken them.

- Place the tablets somewhere you will see them when you need to take them. For example, by your toothbrush, or write little notes to yourself saying **Medication**. Use coloured pieces of paper to remind you if you don't want other people to read your notes.

- Set an alarm on your watch, an alarm clock or the alarm function on a phone to remind you to take tablets at a certain time.

- Ask other people to remind you/phone you if you struggle to remember otherwise.

Please note: All medications can be dangerous if taken in too large a quantity or by mistake. Keep them where young children cannot reach them.

I sometimes take a higher dose than is prescribed

It can be tempting to take extra tablets at times of higher distress to cope, even when your doctor hasn't prescribed the medicine with this in mind. This can cause side effects and is potentially **dangerous.** There can also be unexpected interactions with other medications you take.

KEY POINT

Remember: Taking more tablets than your doctor has prescribed can worsen how you feel. Taking medication at higher than recommended doses may cause unpleasant or dangerous side effects. You get the mistaken idea that you're only managing to cope because of using the medication. You may then come to believe that you can't live life without the medication.

Stopping antidepressants

You may be tempted to stop taking medication without telling your doctor. You may be afraid you are letting them down, or that you will be 'told off' if you do. But it's actually better to discuss any worries you have openly with your doctor. It's important when stopping antidepressants to do it gradually, with a timetable set by your doctor. This reduces the chances of having the possibly severe side effects that can result from stopping the medication too quickly.

>
> **KEY POINT**
> Stopping an antidepressant too early is the most common cause of worsening depression. Many doctors advise their patients to continue to take the antidepressant medication for at least **six months** after they begin to feel better, to prevent slipping back into depression.

Putting things into practice

If you want to find out more about the use of antidepressant medications please discuss this with your doctor. He or she will be able to suggest other sources of information about the treatments that are available.

Summary

In this workbook you have learned:

- How antidepressants are used.
- The answer to some common questions about antidepressants.
- Some useful hints and tips to get the best out of the medication.
- The pros and cons of this type of medication if it is being suggested for you.

Before you go

 What have I learned from this workbook?

 What do I want to try *next*?

Putting into practice what you have learned

Think about what the main issues are for you concerning antidepressant medication. You might need more information, want to discuss starting, changing or stopping medication, or perhaps consider how to better manage side effects.

Suggested reading

Information about recommended treatments for depression is published in various national treatment guidelines. One version that has been written for the general public is available at NICE (**http://publications.nice.org.uk/treating -depression-in-adults-ifp90**).

Plan, Do and Review

Whatever you choose to do, the next step is to do it, and finally to review how things went – whatever happened. The *Planner sheet* and the *Review sheet* are tools to help you do this, and get into a system of *Plan, Do* then *Review* to help you move forward. Copies of both sheets are found at the end of the workbook, and as with all the worksheets can be downloaded from www.llttf.com.

Other sources of support

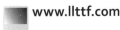 **www.llttf.com**

This popular resource is designed to support readers of this course. There's also a forum where you can make comments or ask questions of other people using the same course.

Acknowledgments

The cartoon illustrations were produced by Keith Chan, kchan75@hotmail.com.

The terms LLTTF and Five Areas are registered trademarks of Five Areas Resources Ltd.

Although we hope you find this book helpful, it's not intended to be a direct substitute for consultative advice with a healthcare professional, nor do we give any assurance about its effectiveness in a particular case. Accordingly, neither the publisher nor the author shall be held liable for any loss or damages arising from its use.

Planner sheet

1. *What* am I going to do?

2. *When* am I going to do it?

Write in the day and time:

3. Is my planned task one that:

Ⓠ Will be useful for helping me move forward?   Yes ☐   No ☐

Ⓠ Is clear, so that I will know when I have done it?   Yes ☐   No ☐

Ⓠ Is something that I value, or need to do?   Yes ☐   No ☐

Ⓠ Is realistic, practical and achievable?   Yes ☐   No ☐

4. What problems/difficulties could arise, and how can I overcome this?

What could get in the way? Write your possible blocks in here:

Do you need to rewrite your plan to tackle these possible blocks?

5. Write down your final plan here

What are you going to do?

When are you going to do it? (day and time)

Your back-up plan: Think of another back-up solution you could turn to if for whatever reason there are problems with your plan.

KEY POINT
If you feel worse with symptoms you can still choose to do the planned activity anyway – because it's important.

Review sheet

What did you plan to do?

Write it here.

What happened? Did you attempt the task?   Yes ☐   No ☐

If yes:

● What went well?

● What didn't go so well?

● What have you learned about from what happened?

● How are you going to apply what you've learned?

If not:
What stopped you?

● *Internal factors* (e.g. forgot, not enough time, put it off, concerns I couldn't do it, I couldn't see the point of it, etc.)

● *External factors* (events that happened, work/home issues, etc.)

● How could you have planned to tackle these blocks?

Use the *Plan, Do, Review* approach to help you move forward.

Overcoming Anxiety, Stress and Panic © Dr Chris Williams 2015

Worksheets to help you practice *Understanding and using antidepressant medication*

Practice is important to help you master this approach. You can download worksheets of all of the key skills used in this workbook from:
www.llttf.com/worksheets/odlm

My notes

Planning for the future

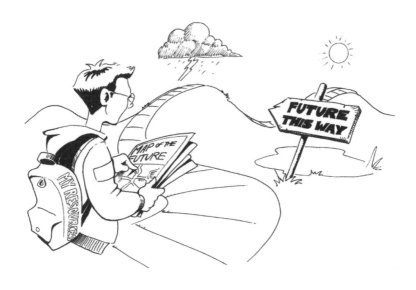

www.llttf.com or www.livinglifetothefull.com @llttfnews (public)

www.fiveareas.com @fiveareas (practitioners)

 www.llttf.com/facebook

Dr Chris Williams

overcoming
depression and low mood
a five areas approach

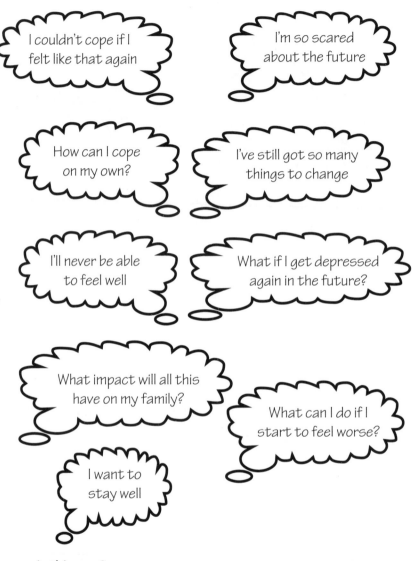

... is this you?

If so... this workbook is for you.

In this workbook you will:

- Look back at what you have learned while working on getting better.
- Summarize key lessons you have learned.
- Work out 'danger signs' that will alert you that you may be slipping back.
- Make a clear plan to stay well.
- Set up some **review days** so you can check your own progress.

The journey of recovery

It can be helpful to think of yourself as being on a **journey of recovery**. In the following sections there are some questions to help you identify **what has helped you** to move on.

My journey

Q What is different now from before?

Q What gains have I made?

Q How have things changed/improved in each of the five areas?

Area 1: Situations, relationships and practical problems

Q How have things changed/improved in the situations and practical problems I face?

Q What practical resources have I discovered in myself and in the support from others around me? (For example, how to build close relationships.)

Area 2: Altered thinking

Q How have things changed/improved in my thinking?

Areas 3 and 4: Altered feelings/physical symptoms and sensations

Q How have things changed/improved in my feelings and the physical symptoms I used to have? (For example, you may still have the same worries and fears, but not be troubled by them as often.)

Area 5: Altered behaviour

Q How have things changed/improved in my behaviour and activity levels? What can I do now and what can't I still do? Do I now respond to things in helpful or unhelpful ways? (For example, have you been more active, faced your fears and done things that you value and give you a sense of pleasure and made you feel close to other people? Are you now more likely to make choices that reflect the person you want to be?)

Working out what's made the difference

 What have I done to make these changes happen?

 What new skills have I gained that I can use to help me continue to improve?

What practical steps can I take to continue making changes?

Some things to do

 Example: Anne's mental fitness plan

- When I begin to feel low and stressed, I need to do something about it before it worsens.
- Don't withdraw from others when I feel down – they can really help me pick up.
- When I feel overwhelmed by problems – just tackle them one at a time.

Task

Now answer the questions in the following table to help make your own plan.

Some things to do	Tick here if this affects your life – even if just sometimes
Tackle things early if you feel worse	
Build on your strengths/resources	☐
Stop, think and reflect on negative thoughts	
Don't let extreme and unhelpful thinking take over	☐
Keep doing things that you boost (that is, those activities that give you value, and give a sense of pleasure, achievement and closeness to other people)	☐
Face up to your fears – don't let avoidance take over	☐
Live reasonably healthily – be active, eating, sleeping – but not obsessively so	☐
Say no – balance demands that you put on yourself Allow space and time for "you"	☐
Use relaxation tapes or techniques if you find them helpful, such as the Anxiety Control Training technique (www.llttf.com)	☐
If you are prescribed an antidepressant medication, take it regularly	☐
Discuss any changes you want to make with your doctor	☐
Letting problems build up and not dealing with them	☐
Letting your thinking spiral out of control	☐
Avoiding things or putting things off; remember the less you do, the worse you feel	☐
Acting in ways that backfire/worsen things (e.g. taking on too much or setting yourself up to fail)	☐
Drinking too much or blocking how you feel by using street drugs	☐

 What else have I learned about getting and staying better?

Staying well: watching out for the problem times

One important thing to do now is watch out for your problem times. If you do this, you can plan in advance what you're going to do if you start to feel worse. This could happen when you suffer any of the following:

- Personal loss: when you feel let down, rejected or abandoned; for example, you lose a friendship or suffer a bereavement.
- Setbacks or challenges; for example illness or unemployment.
- Stress: when you think things are beginning to get out of control. For example, people who have been off work for some time may find it stressful when they first return to work.

 KEY POINT
The key is not to feel that you must avoid these problem times. Instead the challenge is to find ways of tackling them that will help sort out your problem.

Q In which situations am I likely to have setbacks?

Q What do I need to do differently if I encounter these situations?

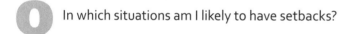

Example: Anne identifies her early warning signs

- ***Situations, relationships and practical problems:*** Feeling overwhelmed by problems and not acting to overcome them.
- ***Altered thinking:*** Becoming very negative and predicting that things will go badly. (negative predictions)
  Having a very negative view of myself (bias against yourself).
  Overlooking good things that happen. (negative mental filter)
  Worrying too much about things that might go wrong (catastrophizing)
- ***Altered feelings:*** Feeling low and weepy, and also feeling very little at all, as though my feelings are becoming numb.

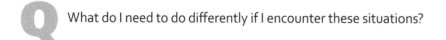

(Continued)

Example: Anne identifies her early warning signs *(Continued)*

- *Altered physical feelings/symptoms:* Feeling very low in energy and finding it hard to get up in the morning. Noticing my sleep pattern worsening.
- *Altered behaviour:* A tendency to want to withdraw and ask my sister not to visit. Stopping doing things I normally enjoy, such as going reading and sitting on the bench in the park. Starting to snack more when I feel stressed.

Anne identifies one key early warning sign:

I am going to watch out for times when I start to avoid people by staying in and not answering the phone.

This key early warning sign means: Do something **now** to tackle how you feel.

Your early warning signs

 Task

Now make your list of early warning signs.
   Area 1: Situations, relationships and practical problems

Overcoming Anxiety, Stress and Panic © Dr Chris Williams 2015

- **Talk to a healthcare practitioner** about your problems and discuss whether you need more help.
- **Choose to stay in contact with people who support you.** Don't isolate yourself – tell others you trust that you are noticing some problems.
- **Respond helpfully.** Keep doing your activities, things that you value and see as important – things that give you a sense of pleasure, achievement or closeness to others. Maintain your healthy helpful habits. Do what has helped you before. Try to make choices that allow you to live your life as you want to.

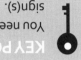

KEY POINT

You need to plan what you will do in response to your key early warning sign(s).

You may watch as if there was no problem? Or do you keep watching TV and keep watching TV. What do you do? Do you ignore it and keep watching TV as if there was no problem? Or do you get up to deal with it?

Imagine one day you hear a smoke alarm bleeping while you're watching TV. What

Making an emergency plan

My **key** early warning sign(s):

Area 5: Altered behaviour/activity levels

Area 4: Altered physical symptoms/sensations

Area 3: Altered feelings/emotions

Area 2: Altered thinking

- Create an **emergency plan** to help you to tackle any early warning signs you notice. The following example shows how Anne decides to react to her early warning signs.

 Example: Anne's early warning sign emergency plan

Altered thinking: with negative predictions and mind-reading	I need to identify and challenge extreme and unhelpful thinking
Altered feelings: feeling low and weepy	Do all the above things, and also go to see my doctor to talk about whether other help or support may be useful
Altered physical symptoms: feeling low in energy, and worse in the morning	Plan to do more difficult tasks later on in the day. Do things at a reasonable pace
Altered behaviour: withdrawing from doing things I like	Create an action plan to do things that give me a sense of pleasure and achievement
Altered behaviour: asking my sister not to visit	Choose to ask Mary to come over each week for a short period of time

Your emergency response plan

Q What is your **emergency plan** in case you have a setback?

Try to be very clear about the things you could do. Include your own mental fitness plan as well as any people you could contact to ask for help. Going back to the example of the smoke alarm, if a fire was getting worse at home in spite of your attempts to tackle it, you would call for professional help. Similarly, if you feel worse in spite of your emergency plan, you should get in touch with someone who can help. They can advise you whether other approaches may be helpful.

Plan a regular review day

Every week, choose a day in your calendar as a 'review' day. If this seems too often, try to do this at least once a month – perhaps on the last day of the month, so you can look back over recent weeks. During this **review** time, try to spend 30 minutes or so thinking back over things since your last review.

Here are some ideas about how to go about your review.

- Complete a blank Five Areas assessment (there's one at the end of this workbook). Check how you are doing in each area. Any progress? Any setbacks? Do you need to re-read or work on any new areas? Do you need extra advice/help?

- What's gone well and less well? Look back over your plans and how they have gone. Use your *Planner* and *Review sheets* to do this (again at the end of this workbook).

- Are you slipping back (review your warning signs list or emergency plan if needed)?

- What can you learn from what has happened?

- How can you put what has been learned into practice?

My plan for the next few weeks (consider short-, medium- and long-term changes):

Now, based on this review, think about your plans over the next few weeks and months. Consider short-, medium- and long-term targets.

Planning for the future

What are you going to do next?

Do you need to break those targets down into smaller steps?

Once you have a clear first target, write a plan using the *Planner sheet* to plan this next step. You can then review how you do using the *Review sheet*. Copies of both are at the end of this workbook and can be obtained also from www.llttf.com.

> **KEY POINT**
> The important thing is to commit yourself to Plan, Do and Review regularly over the long term.

Sources of extra help

- **Your family doctor/physician.** Your doctor can offer medical advice and (if they feel it is necessary) refer you to a mental health specialist for a detailed assessment.
- **Social services.** Social services can be a great source of support for families. You can find your local social services office hours' enquiry phone number and a 24-hour emergency phone number in local directories or online.

Summary
In this workbook you have:

1. Looked back at what you have learned.
2. Identified the key lessons you have learned.
3. Learned about your 'danger signs' that tell you things may be slipping back.
4. Learned how to make a clear plan to stay well.
5. Set up a regular pattern of Plan, Do and Review, so **you can check** your progress. Use the *Planner* and *Review sheets* to help you do this.
6. Use the idea of a review day to look back on your overall progress and set new short-, medium- and longer-term targets.

Before you go

What have I learned from this workbook?

What do I want to try next?

Putting into practice what you have learned

You are likely to make the most progress and build on the progress you have made if you keep putting into practice what you have learned about improving how you feel. This workbook contains various suggestions – a plan to cope, watching for signs you are slipping back, and creating an emergency plan.

Suggested task

Pick one of those areas and use the *Planner sheet* to make a plan to do it.

Whatever you choose to do, try to maintain the underlying pattern of Plan, Do and Review throughout the week and month. Keep reflecting on how things are going, giving yourself a pat on the back when things go well, and being gentle on yourself if you have a setback. Remember you're not on your own, many millions of people experience low mood at some time in life, and through courses like this, support online, through families and friends as well as through healthcare professionals, help is at hand.

Other sources of support

1. www.llttf.com (www.livinglifetothefull.com; **@llttfnews)**
This popular resource is designed to support readers of this course. There's also a forum where you can make comments or ask questions of other people using the same course.

2. www.llttfshop.com for Five Areas resources and books (for the public).

3. www.fiveareas.com (**@fiveareas.com** for practitioner support and training).

Other resources

Here are some other Five Areas resources that can be helpful at times of low or anxious mood:

- *24 hours to get a job that really fires you up.* (Highly Commended BMA book awards 2013) (Kindle)
- *Overcoming anxiety: a Five Areas approach.*
- *Are you strong enough to keep your temper?* (Kindle)
- *I'm not good enough (low confidence).* (Kindle)
- *Stop smoking in 5 minutes.* (Kindle)
- *I feel so bad I can't go on.* (Highly Commended BMA book awards 2013) (Kindle)
- *Fix your drinking problem in 2 days.* (Kindle) (Linked website at www.littf4drink.com)
- *Enjoy your baby* (postnatal depression). (Kindle)
- *Reclaim your life from illness, disability, pain or fatigue.* (Kindle)
- *I'm not supposed to feel like this: a Christian self-help approach to depression and anxiety,* C. Williams, P. Richards and I. Whitton. (A linked website is at www.littfwg.com)

A request for feedback

Finally, you've finished this course. Well done! I hope it's been helpful. The content of the Five Areas courses is updated and improved on a regular basis based on feedback from users and practitioners. If there are areas in the workbooks that you found hard to understand, or that seemed unclear or confusing, please let me know. However, please note that I cannot provide specific advice on treatment.

To provide feedback please contact us:

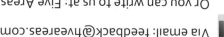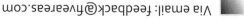

Via email: feedback@fiveareas.com

Or you can write to us at: Five Areas, PO Box 9, Glasgow G63 0WL, UK

In your feedback, please state which workbook, book or website you are commenting on.

Acknowledgments

The cartoon illustrations were produced by Keith Chan, kchan75@hotmail.com. The *Planner and Review sheets,* and *Plan, Do, Review* model are reproduced from the Living Life to the Full course courtesy of Five Areas Resources Ltd© (2009–2013).

The terms LLTTF and Five Areas are registered trademarks of Five Areas Resources Ltd.

Planner sheet

1. *What am I going to do?*

_____

2. *When am I going to do it?*
Write in the day and time:

3. Is my planned task one that:

🔑 Will be useful for helping me move forward?	☐ Yes	☐ No
🔑 Is clear, so that I will know when I have done it?	☐ Yes	☐ No
🔑 Is something that I value, or need to do?	☐ Yes	☐ No
🔑 Is realistic, practical and achievable?	☐ Yes	☐ No

4. What problems/difficulties could arise, and how can I overcome this?
What could get in the way? Write your possible blocks in here:

Do you need to re-write your plan to tackle these possible blocks?

5. Write down your final plan here
What are you going to do?

When are you going to do it? (day and time)

Your back-up plan: Think of another back-up solution you could turn to if for whatever reason there are problems with your plan.

> 🔑 **KEY POINT**
> If you feel worse with symptoms you can still choose to do the planned
> activity anyway – because it's important.

Planning for the future

Review sheet

What did you plan to do?

Write it here.

What happened? Did you attempt the task?   Yes ☐   No ☐

If yes:

- What went well?

- What didn't go so well?

- What have you learned about from what happened?

- How are you going to apply what you've learned?

If not:

What stopped you?

- *Internal factors* (e.g. forgot, not enough time, put it off, concerns I couldn't do it, I couldn't see the point of it, etc.)

- *External factors* (events that happened, work/home issues, etc.)

- How could you have planned to tackle these blocks?

Use the *Plan, Do, Review* approach to help you move forward.

Planning for the future

Worksheets to help you practice *Planning for the future*

Practice is important to help you master this approach. You can download worksheets of all of the key skills used in this workbook from:

www.llttf.com/worksheets/odlm

My notes